Differential Diagnoses in Surgical Pathology:
Breast

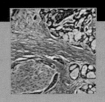 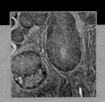 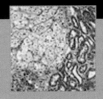 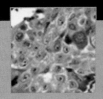
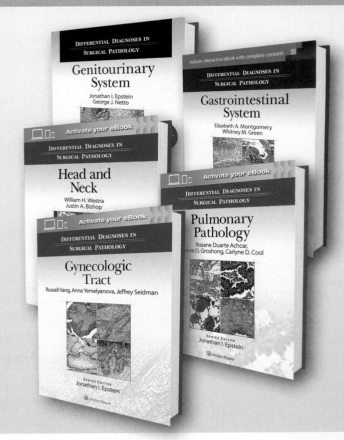
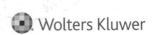

Differential Diagnoses in Surgical Pathology:
Breast

Jean F. Simpson, MD

President
Breast Pathology Consultants, Inc.
Nashville, Tennessee
Adjunct Professor of Pathology
University of South Alabama
Mobile, Alabama

Melinda E. Sanders, MD

Professor of Pathology, Microbiology, and Immunology
Vanderbilt University Medical Center
Nashville, Tennessee

SERIES EDITOR

Jonathan I. Epstein, MD

Professor of Pathology, Urology and Oncology
The Reinhard Professor of Urological Pathology
Director of Surgical Pathology
The Johns Hopkins Medical Institutions
Baltimore, Maryland

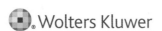

. Wolters Kluwer

Philadelphia • Baltimore • New York • London
Buenos Aires • Hong Kong • Sydney • Tokyo

Acquisitions Editor: Ryan Shaw
Product Development Editor: Kate Heaney
Production Project Manager: Alicia Jackson
Manufacturing Coordinator: Beth Welsh
Marketing Manager: Dan Dressler
Design Coordinator: Teresa Mallon
Production Service: S4Carlisle Publishing Services

9 8 7 6 5 4 3 2 1

Printed in China

Library of Congress Cataloging-in-Publication Data
Names: Simpson, Jean F., author. | Sanders, Melinda E., author.
Title: Breast/Jean F. Simpson, Melinda E. Sanders.
Other titles: Differential diagnoses in surgical pathology series.
Description: Philadelphia: Wolters Kluwer Health, [2017] | Series:
  Differential diagnoses in surgical pathology | Includes bibliographical
  references and index.
Identifiers: LCCN 2016038688 | ISBN 9781496300652
Subjects: | MESH: Breast Neoplasms—diagnosis | Breast Neoplasms—pathology |
  Diagnosis, Differential | Pathology, Surgical--methods
Classification: LCC RC280.B8 | NLM WP 870 | DDC 616.99/449—dc23 LC record available at https://lccn.loc.gov/2016038688

DEDICATION

In memory of Lowell W. Rogers and J. Allan Tucker, gentle giants who inspired others.

PREFACE

Histopathology remains the cornerstone of the diagnosis and treatment of breast disease. There have been advances in breast imaging techniques, molecular analysis, and immunotherapy of breast cancer, yet the fundamental decisions regarding the need for additional surgery, chemoprevention, radiation, and/or chemotherapy are based on morphologic features.

Histopathology is far from a static or "out of date" discipline. Indeed, specific histologic criteria have been defined that allow for reproducibility in diagnosis; linking these criteria to outcome data for thousands of women through long-term follow-up studies has defined the epidemiology of benign breast disease and helps identify women who may benefit from chemoprevention strategies. These studies also provide concrete evidence that merely undergoing a breast biopsy does not increase risk for later cancer development, a welcome relief for thousands of women.

The widespread use of core needle biopsy has had a major impact on the practice of breast pathology, and many of the images shown in this book are from core needle biopsy specimens. Our approach to the diagnosis of core biopsy specimens is similar to a frozen section, that is, what should the next step be, specifically, should the lesion be formally excised?

We are grateful for the opportunity to have learned breast pathology from Dr. David Page, whose adherence to reproducible criteria and interpretation within the clinical context guide us daily. We also are grateful to pathologists who have trusted us with their difficult cases in consultation. The vast majority of such cases come with a differential diagnosis of one or two entities, underscoring the importance of a textbook that compares and contrasts differential diagnostic partners.

Jean F. Simpson
Melinda E. Sanders

CONTENTS

1

Nonproliferative Alterations of Acini

	Columnar Cell Lesion without Atypia	Cystically Dilated Lobular Unit
Age	Adult women	Adult women
Imaging findings	Calcifications, punctuate in clusters	Calcification or lobulated mass, often with septations
Etiology	Unknown	Unknown change in specialized connective tissue results in unfolding of the lobular unit
Histology	1. Lobular unit is enlarged 2. Lined by columnar cells that maintain basolateral polarity *(Figs. 1.1.1–1.1.3)*	Unfolded, coalescing acini, lined by a single epithelial cell layer, usually cuboidal or apocrine *(Figs. 1.1.4–1.1.6)*
Special studies	None	None
Treatment	None	Fine needle aspiration if symptomatic
Clinical implication	No risk implications	No risk implications

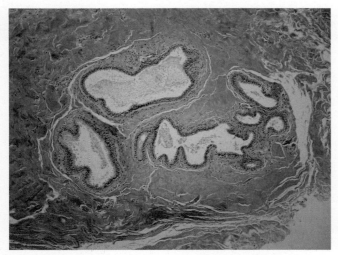

Figure 1.1.1   Columnar cell lesion without atypia: The lobular unit is enlarged and consists of dilated acini with undulating contours. The intra-lobular connective tissue is fibrotic.

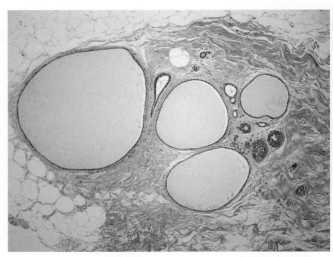

Figure 1.1.4   Cystically dilated lobular unit: Half of the acini of this lobular unit are expanded, but maintain rounded contours.

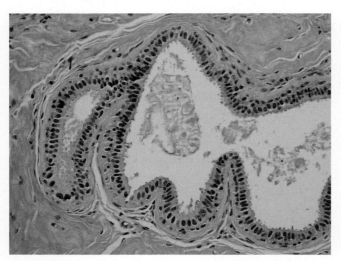

Figure 1.1.2   The dilated acini contain secretions and are lined by a single layer of columnar cells; the relationship with the myoepithelial cell layer is orderly in columnar cell lesions without atypia.

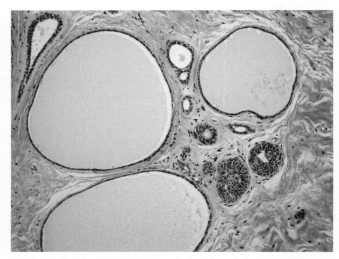

Figure 1.1.5   The dilated acini contain translucent secretions and lack histiocyes or inflammatory cells. Acini of normal size and configuration are present adjacent to the dilated acini.

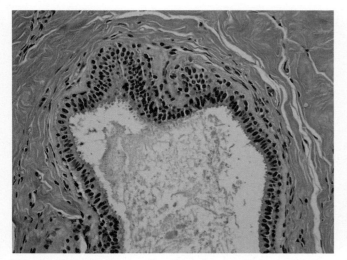

Figure 1.1.3   The columnar cells maintain basolateral polarity. Nuclei are small, without obvious nucleoli. The myoepithelial cells are prominent.

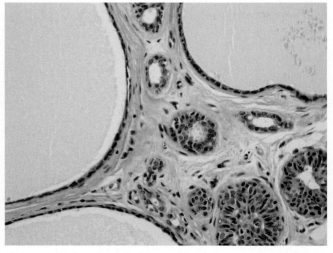

Figure 1.1.6   The cystically dilated acini are lined by a single layer of normally polarized, low cuboidal epithelium, with patchy attenuation.

	Columnar Cell Lesion without Atypia	Columnar Cell Lesion with Atypia
Age	Adult women	Adult women
Imaging findings	Calcifications, typically in clusters, usually punctate, may be amorphous, rarely pleomorphic	Calcifications, typically in clusters, may be punctate or amorphous, rarely pleomorphic
Etiology	Unknown	Unknown
Histology	1. Enlarged lobular unit lined by one or two cell layers 2. Maintenance of basolateral polarity 3. Nuclei lack prominent nucleoli *(Figs. 1.2.1–1.2.5)*	1. Enlarged lobular units lined by epithelial cells that have lost basolateral polarity 2. Rounded nuclei often with prominent nucleolus *(Figs. 1.2.6–1.2.10)* 3. Lacks architectural features of atypical ductal hyperplasia (ADH), e.g., Cribriform spaces or micropapillae
Genetic abnormalities	None	Loss of chromosome 16q
Treatment	Excision unnecessary if detected on core biopsy	Excision if present in core biopsy specimen because of association with more clinically significant lesions; no treatment necessary if detected in excisional biopsy specimen
Clinical implication	None	Slight increase in relative cancer risk (1.5×)

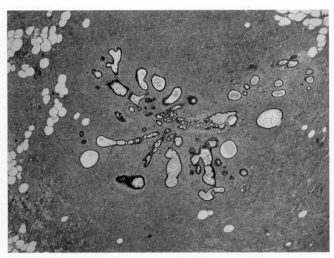

Figure 1.2.1 Columnar cell lesion without atypia. Most acini in the lobular unit are enlarged and have irregular contours.

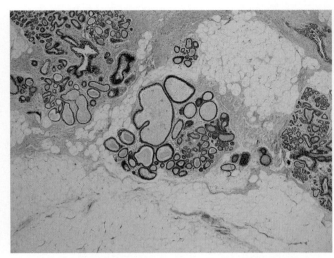

Figure 1.2.6 Columnar cell lesion with atypia: Two adjacent lobular units contain several enlarged, dilated acini. At low power, the character of the lining cells is not evident.

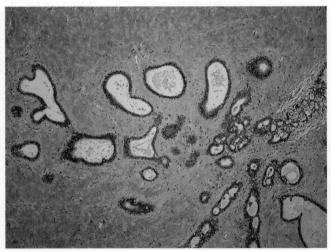

Figure 1.2.2 The enlarged acini contain calcifying secretions and a single columnar luminal epithelial cell layer.

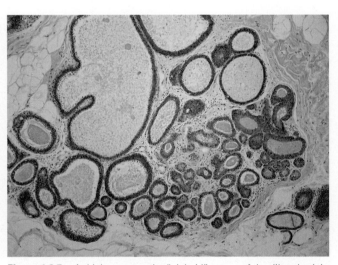

Figure 1.2.7 At higher power, the "globoid" nature of the dilated acini is evident in columnar cell lesions with atypia.

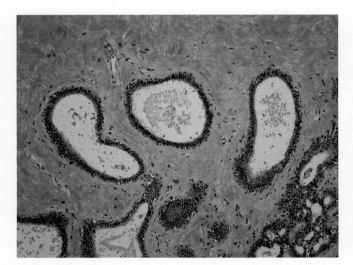

Figure 1.2.3 The acinar cells are distinctly elongated and have prominent apical snouts.

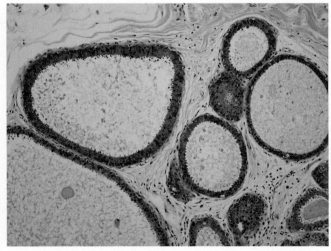

Figure 1.2.8 Columnar cell lesion with atypia: These dilated acini contain secretions and are lined by cells with rounded nuclei with an increased nuclear to cytoplasmic ratio.

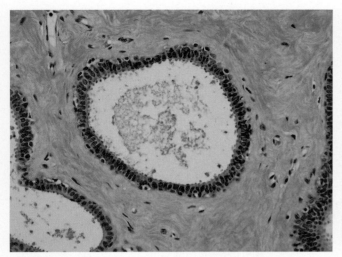

Figure 1.2.4 The columnar lining cells maintain normal basolateral polarity. The myoepithelial layer is regularly identifiable.

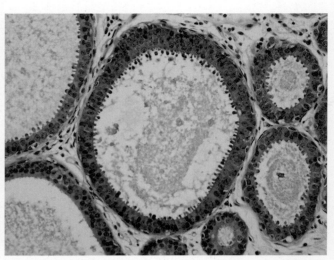

Figure 1.2.9 The acini are lined by several layers of luminal epithelial cells with loss of a polar arrangement. Myoepithelial cells are present, but not prominent. Apocrine snouts are observed in most acini. Note the conspicuous absence of architectural features diagnostic of ADH i.e., cribriform spaces, bars, or bulbous papillae.

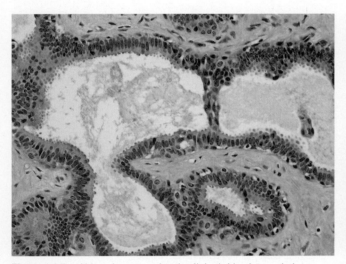

Figure 1.2.5 Although an occasional cellular bridge is noted, the nuclei are overlapping with their long axes oriented parallel with the bar, diagnostic criterion for usual hyperplasia. Focal pseudostratification or tangential sectioning may create the appearance of multiple cell layers and loss of polarity.

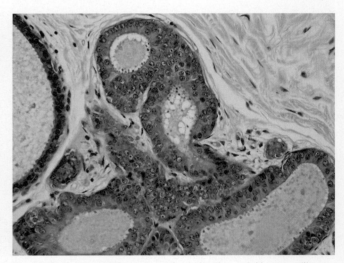

Figure 1.2.10 In addition to loss of polarity, the nuclei have readily apparent nucleoli; compare with the adjacent acinus lined by a single layer of smaller nuclei (left side).

	Apocrine Change	Columnar Cell Lesion with Atypia
Age	Adult women	Adult women
Imaging findings	"Milk of calcium" type calcifications may be present in clusters; aggregated apocrine cysts may form a mass with associated calcifications	Calcifications typically in clusters, may be punctate, amorphous, or rarely pleomorphic
Clinical associations	Often perimenopausal	No specific associations
Histology	1. Dilated lobular unit *(Fig. 1.3.1)*, lined by a single layer of apocrine cells *(Fig. 1.3.2)* 2. May have apical red cytoplasmic granules 3. Nuclei enlarged with prominent nucleolus *(Figs. 1.3.3 and 1.3.4)*	1. Enlarged lobular units lined by epithelial cells that have lost normal basolateral polarity 2. Crowded, rounded, enlarged nuclei, often with a prominent nucleolus 3. Lacks architectural features of ADH, e.g., Cribriform spaces or micropapillae *(Figs. 1.3.5–1.3.8)*
Genetic abnormalities	None	Loss of chromosome 16q
Treatment	Cyst drainage by fine needle aspiration	Excision if present in core biopsy specimen because of association with other more clinically significant lesions; no further treatment necessary if detected in excisional biopsy specimen
Clinical implication	No increase in cancer risk	1.5× increased relative cancer risk of subsequent breast cancer

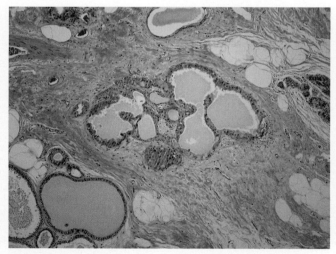

Figure 1.3.1 Apocrine change involving two adjacent lobular units. Acini have partially coalesced, and contain eosinophilic secretory material.

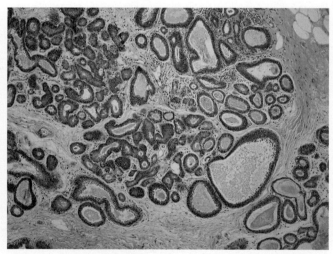

Figure 1.3.5 Columnar cell lesion with atypia: Three adjacent lobular units are expanded with variably sized acini; pronounced basophilia reflects an increased nuclear to cytoplasmic ratio.

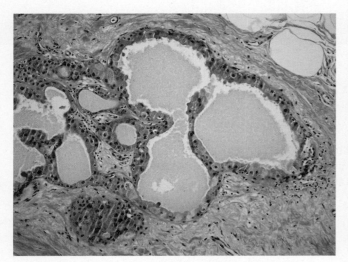

Figure 1.3.2   Apocrine change composed of dilated acini lined by a single layer of cuboidal cells.

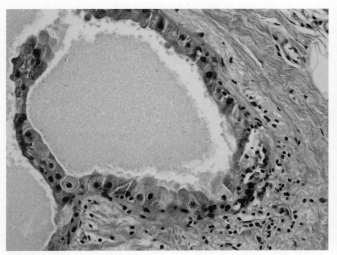

Figure 1.3.3   Apocrine cytoplasm is abundant, pale to eosinophilic, and finely granular. A normal nuclear to cytoplasmic ratio is maintained.

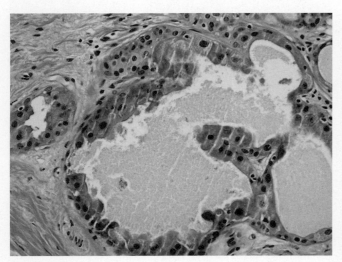

Figure 1.3.4   Bland-appearing, rounded nuclei are characteristic, and normal polarity is maintained. The apical compartment of the cytoplasm contains characteristic red granules.

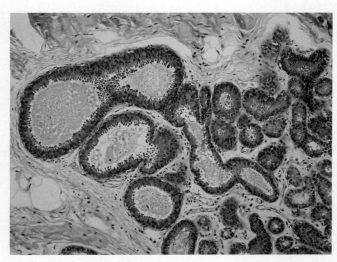

Figure 1.3.6   Dilated acini are lined by columnar cells with prominent apocrine snouts. Nuclear enlargement and lack of the normal basolateral polarity are evident at this magnification.

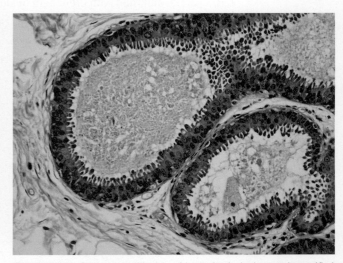

Figure 1.3.7   Columnar cell lesion with atypia: A single pseudostratified cell layer shows "rounding up" of nuclei. Myoepithelial cells are present, but not prominent. There are no complex architectural arrangements to suggest ADH.

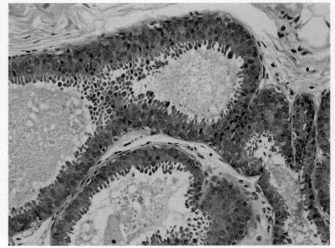

Figure 1.3.8   Tangential sectioning may give the appearance of multilayering. Focally, the apical snouts are apposed, but there are no true arches or bridging.

	Secretory Change	Columnar Cell Lesion with Atypia
Age	Any age, usually women in reproductive years	Any age, predominantly 40–60 y
Imaging findings	Clustered mammographic calcifications, usually spherical	Clustered mammographic calcifications, may be punctate, amorphous or rarely pleomorphic
Clinical associations	Often present postlactation; prolactin-producing pituitary tumors; drugs causing prolactin secretion	Unknown
Histology	1. All or part of a lobular unit may show secretory change *(Fig. 1.4.1)* 2. Acini are variably dilated *(Fig. 1.4.2)* and lined by cells that have eosinophilic, bubbly cytoplasm 3. Secretory material is present in lumens *(Fig. 1.4.2)* 4. Cells contain small dark nuclei with a hobnail appearance *(Fig. 1.4.3)* 5. Nuclei are in the apical compartment, similar to the Arias-Stella reaction *(Fig. 1.4.3)*	1. Enlarged basophilic lobular units, with a "globoid configuration," having variably dilated acini *(Fig. 1.4.4)* 2. Lumens contain secretory material which is frequently calcified *(Fig. 1.4.5)* 3. Acini are lined by cells lacking basolateral polarity *(Figs. 1.4.6 and 1.4.7)* 4. Nuclei are round, and have prominent nucleoli *(Fig. 1.4.7)* 5. Apical snouts are common *(Fig. 1.4.8)*
Genetic abnormalities	None	Loss of chromosome 16q
Treatment	None	Excisional biopsy if present in core needle biopsy because of association with other clinically significant lesions; no further treatment if present in an excisional specimen
Clinical implication	None	1.5× increased relative risk of subsequent breast cancer

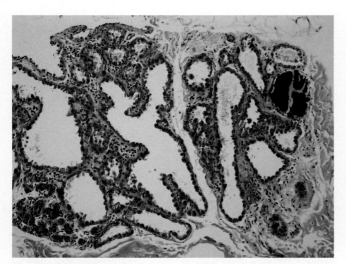

Figure 1.4.1 Secretory change partially involving two adjacent lobular units, characterized by several dilated acini, one of which has undulating contours. Note the spherical calcification (right). The lobular unit in the bottom left contains several normal acini.

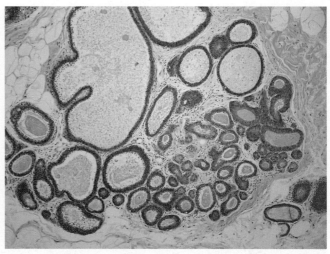

Figure 1.4.4 Columnar cell lesion with atypia: Note the globoid configuration of the acini in this enlarged lobular unit; most contain secretory material within their lumens.

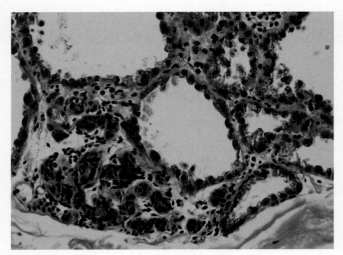

Figure 1.4.2 Acini lined by a single layer of cuboidal cells with eosinophilic, "bubbly" inclusions characterizes secretory change.

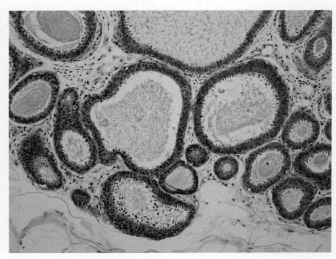

Figure 1.4.5 Prominent basophilia is a hallmark of columnar cell lesions with atypia.

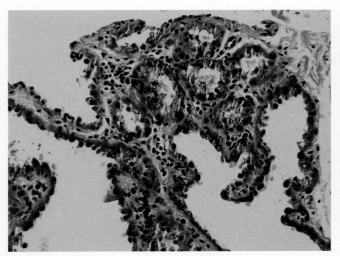

Figure 1.4.3 The nuclei in secretory change are dark, have a "smudged" appearance, and are present in the apical compartment ("hobnail" cells), similar to the Arias-Stella cytologic change of the endometrium.

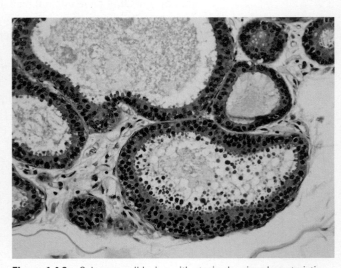

Figure 1.4.6 Columnar cell lesion with atypia showing characteristic nuclear enlargement, "rounding up," and loss of polarity.

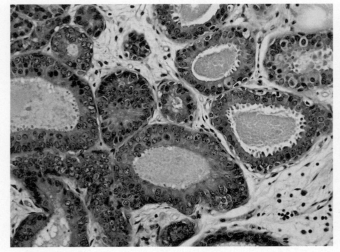

Figure 1.4.7 Columnar cell lesion with atypia showing loss of cellular polarity, nuclear enlargement, and prominent nucleoli. Myoepithelial cells are present.

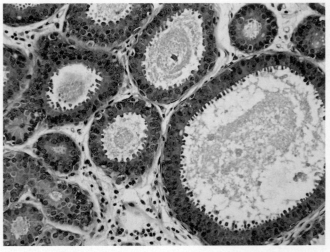

Figure 1.4.8 Nucleoli are also evident in this example of columnar cell lesion with atypia, although not as pronounced as in Figure 1.4.7.

	Cystically Dilated Lobular Unit	Duct Ectasia
Age	Perimenopausal	Peri- or postmenopausal
Imaging findings	Calcifications, or rounded mass often with septations	Dilated lactiferous ducts containing inspissated secretions; branching calcifications. Pattern on mammogram is quite specific
Etiology	Unknown	Unknown, occasionally present following mastitis, or in smokers
Histology	1. Unfolded, coalescing acini results in cyst formation 2. Architecture of lobular unit may not be obvious *(Fig. 1.5.1)* 3. Cyst lining may be attenuated *(Fig. 1.5.2)*, or cuboidal *(Fig. 1.5.3)* 4. Foamy histiocytes are frequently present in lumens *(Fig. 1.5.4)* 5. With longstanding cysts, there may be pericystic fibrosis, but no duct wall is present *(Fig. 1.5.4)*	1. Disease of true ducts 2. Dilated ducts containing inspissated grumous material, periductal fibrosis and chronic inflammation *(Figs. 1.5.5–1.5.8)*
Genetic abnormalities	None	None
Treatment	Fine needle aspiration if symptomatic	None
Clinical implication	No cancer risk implications	No cancer risk implications

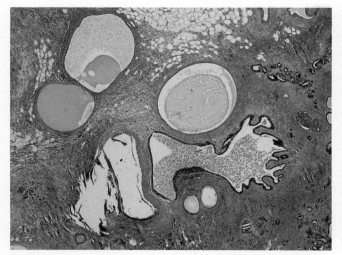

Figure 1.5.1 Cystically dilated lobular unit: Acini have unfolded and coalesced.

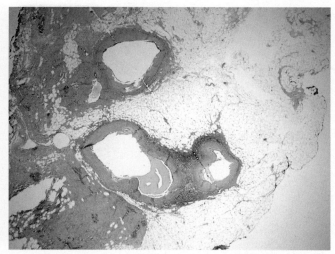

Figure 1.5.5 Duct ectasia characterized by thickly fibrotic duct walls and brisk periductal chronic inflammation.

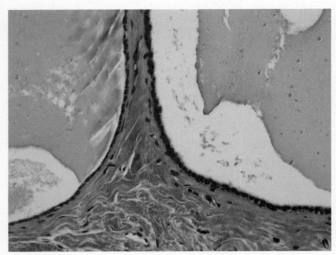

Figure 1.5.2 This cystically dilated lobular unit is lined by a single layer of low cuboidal epithelium. The specialized connective tissue of the lobular unit is replaced by fibrotic stroma, but there is no duct wall surrounding the enlarged space.

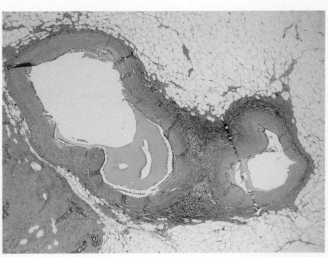

Figure 1.5.6 Duct ectasia: The contours of this fibrotic structure are characteristic of a true duct. Note grumous material within the lumen and marked attenuation/focal absence of the epithelium lining this duct.

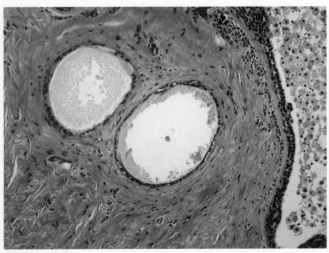

Figure 1.5.3 In addition to luminal histiocytes within this cyst, occasional histiocytes are intermixed in the lining epithelium. The adjacent smaller cysts contain secretions only.

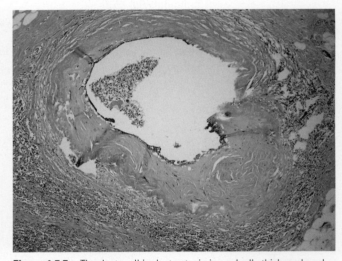

Figure 1.5.7 The duct wall in duct ectasia is markedly thickened, and there is a prominent rind of periductal chronic inflammation.

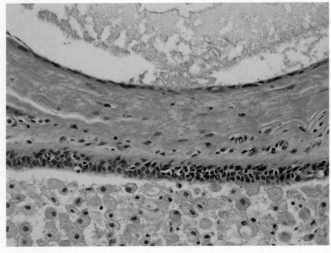

Figure 1.5.4 A simple cyst is lined by attenuated epithelium (top), while an adjacent cyst maintains a two-cell layer and contains numerous foamy histiocytes (bottom).

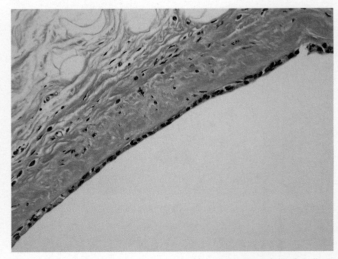

Figure 1.5.8 Duct ectasia showing marked attenuation of the duct lining epithelium.

	Mucocele-Like Lesion	Disrupted Cyst
Age	Adult women	Adult women
Imaging findings	Calcifications, or rounded mass	Calcifications
Etiology	Unknown	Unknown
Histology	1. Rupture of terminal duct lobular unit with pools of mucin insinuating into stroma 2. Residual epithelial cells may be loosely attached to the preexisting wall of the dilated space *(Figs. 1.6.1–1.6.8)*	1. Rounded contour of cyst remains 2. Cyst lining is often obliterated and cyst contents, foamy histiocytes and giant cells, become admixed with stromal cells immediately adjacent to the cyst, without dissection into the stroma *(Figs. 1.6.9–1.6.12)*
Genetic abnormalities	None	None
Treatment	Excision required only if associated with another lesion that requires excision, i.e., ADH	None
Clinical implication	Mucocele-like lesion may be associated with cysts, usual hyperplasia, atypical hyperplasia, ductal carcinoma in situ, or mucinous carcinoma. Associated epithelial changes dictate the risk implication.	None

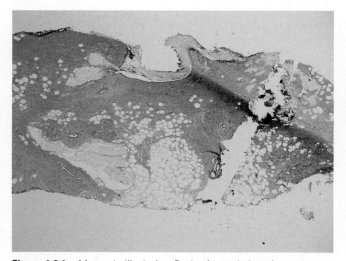

Figure 1.6.1 Mucocele-like lesion: Pools of extruded mucin are present in nonspecialized connective tissue adjacent to a disrupted duct and a large, dystrophic calcification.

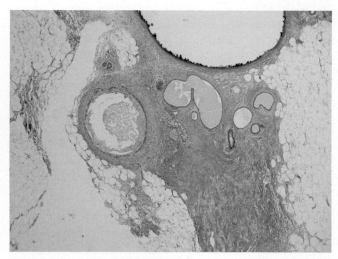

Figure 1.6.9 Apocrine cysts showing rupture. The cyst contains basophilic secretory material, not mucin.

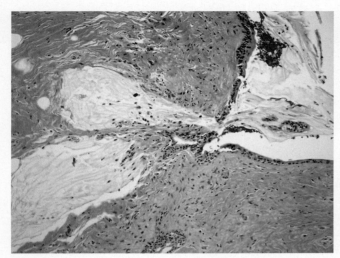

Figure 1.6.2   The mucin pools adjacent to the disrupted cyst contain a few bland, degenerated epithelial elements.

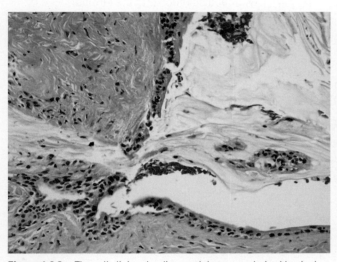

Figure 1.6.3   The cells lining the disrupted duct are polarized luminal epithelial cells with abundant cytoplasm and round basally located nuclei. A prominent myoepithelial layer is also present (bottom).

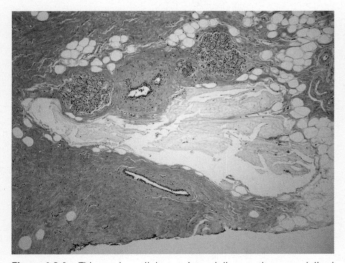

Figure 1.6.4   This nearly acellular mucin pool dissects the unspecialized connective tissue.

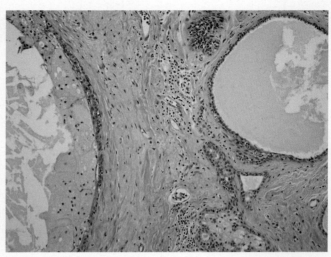

Figure 1.6.10   Foamy histiocytes are present within this cyst (left), as well as in the surrounding stroma.

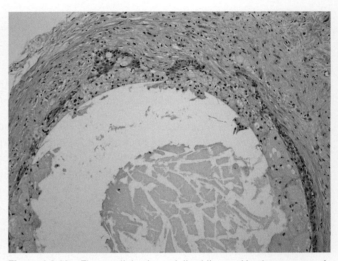

Figure 1.6.11   The cyst lining is partially obliterated by the presence of foamy histiocytes; some are also present in the adjacent stroma.

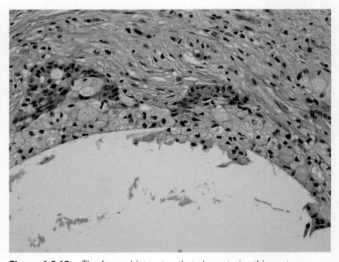

Figure 1.6.12   The foamy histocytes that characterize this cyst can mimic epithelium with clear cell change or intracytoplasmic mucin.

1.6 Mucocele-Like Lesion vs. Disrupted Cyst **15**

1 Nonproliferative

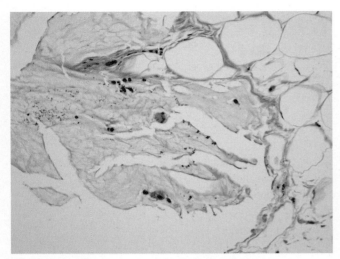

Figure 1.6.5   A few degenerated epithelial cells are noted in the extravasated mucin in this mucocele-like lesion.

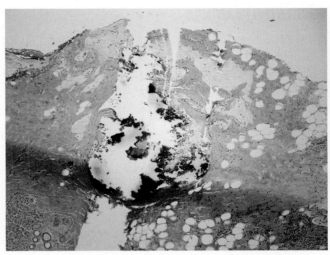

Figure 1.6.6   The large, fractured calcification fills an enlarged duct. The surrounding stroma contains multiple small mucin pools characteristic of a mucocele-like lesion.

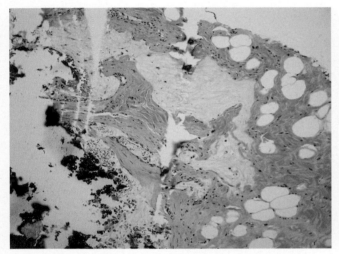

Figure 1.6.7   The distorted duct filled with calcifications has a barely detectable, attenuated lining in this mucocele-like lesion.

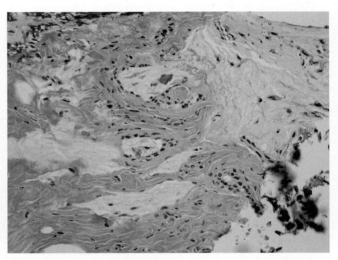

Figure 1.6.8   The few cellular elements in the extravasated mucin are degenerated in this mucocele-like lesion.

SUGGESTED READINGS

Aroner SA, Collins LC, Schnitt SJ, et al. Columnar cell lesions and subsequent breast cancer risk: a nested case–control study. *Breast Cancer Res.* 2010;12:R61.

Boulos FI, Dupont WD, Simpson JF, et al. Histologic associations and long-term cancer risk in columnar cell lesions of the breast: a retrospective cohort and a nested case–control study. *Cancer.* 2008;113:2415–2421.

Dupont WD, Page DL. Risk factors for breast cancer in women with proliferative breast disease. *N Engl J Med.* 1985;312:146–151.

Hartmann LC, Sellers TA, Frost MH, et al. Benign breast disease and the risk of breast cancer. *N Engl J Med.* 2005;353:229–237.

London SJ, Connolly JL, Schnitt SJ, et al. A prospective study of benign breast disease and the risk of breast cancer. *JAMA.* 1992;267:941–944.

Rosen PP. Columnar cell hyperplasia is associated with lobular carcinoma in situ and tubular carcinoma. *Am J Surg Pathol.* 1999;23:1561.

Sahoo S, Recant WM. Triad of columnar cell alteration, lobular carcinoma in situ, and tubular carcinoma of the breast. *Breast J.* 2005;11:140–142.

Schnitt SJ, Collins LC. Columnar cell lesions and flat epithelial atypia of the breast. *Semin Breast Dis.* 2005:100–111.

Schnitt SJ, Vincent-Salomon A. Columnar cell lesions of the breast. *Adv Anat Pathol.* 2003;10:113–124.

2

Epithelial Proliferative Lesions, Usual and Atypical Ductal Hyperplasia

	Florid Hyperplasia without Atypia	Cribriform-Pattern Atypical Ductal Hyperplasia (ADH)
Age	Adult women	Adult women
Imaging findings	Calcifications, rarely mass, often incidental	Calcifications, often incidental
Etiology	Unknown	Unknown
Histology	1. Affects terminal duct lobular unit *(Fig. 2.1.1)* 2. Nuclear variability and overlap *(Figs. 2.1.1–2.1.5)* 3. Irregular secondary spaces *(Figs. 2.1.2–2.1.5)* 4. Indistinct cell borders *(Figs. 2.1.4 and 2.1.5)*	1. Affects terminal duct lobular unit *(Figs. 2.1.6 and 2.1.7)* 2. Uniform cell population with even cell placement *(Figs. 2.1.8 and 2.1.9)* 3. Distinct cell borders; solid pattern of ADH shows microrosette formation with cells evenly arranged around small lumens *(Figs. 2.1.8 and 2.1.9)*
Special studies	None; CK5/6 is variably expressed	None; CK5/6 is usually not expressed
Genetic abnormalities	None	Loss of 16q, 17p
Treatment	None	Excision if detected in core biopsy specimen; mammographic follow-up ± antiestrogen therapy
Clinical implication	Slightly increased risk of later cancer development (1.5×); risk level insufficient to affect patient management	Moderately increased risk of later cancer development (4–5×); risk is bilateral

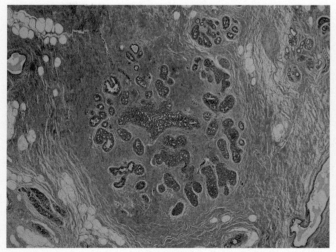

Figure 2.1.1 Florid hyperplasia without atypia: A terminal duct lobular unit is expanded by proliferating epithelial cells; the proliferation is confined to the lobular unit without involving an adjacent true duct.

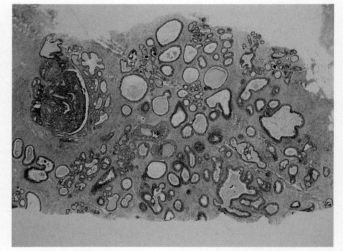

Figure 2.1.6 ADH: Several lobular units have dilated acini that show epithelial hyperplasia.

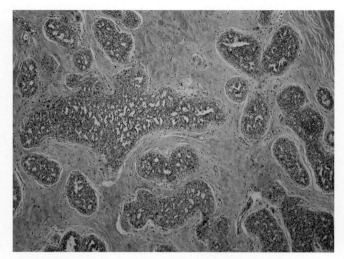

Figure 2.1.2   The secondary spaces created by the epithelial hyperplasia have an irregular shape.

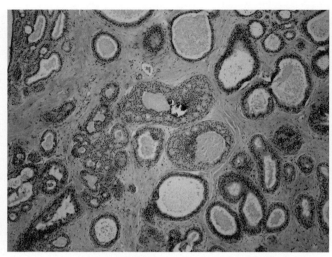

Figure 2.1.7   The two acini in the center contain a proliferation of epithelial cells; secondary spaces are peripheral but uniform in this example of ADH. Microcalcifications are present in one of the involved acini.

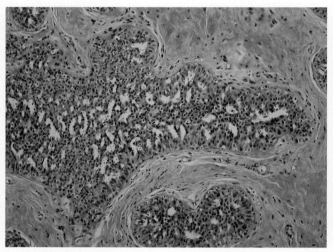

Figure 2.1.3   Secondary spaces are fenestrated and not sharply defined in florid hyperplasia without atypia.

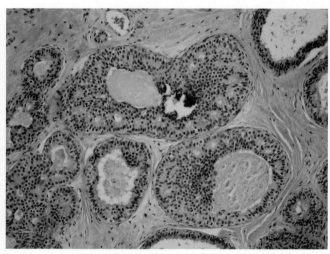

Figure 2.1.8   Nuclear uniformity and even cell placement characterize ADH.

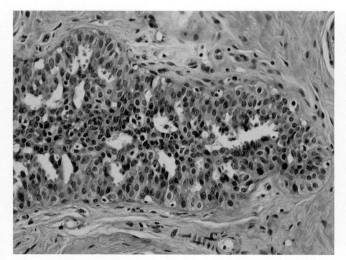

Figure 2.1.4   The irregular secondary spaces are a manifestation of uneven cell placement; note nuclear variability and overlap in this example of florid hyperplasia without atypia.

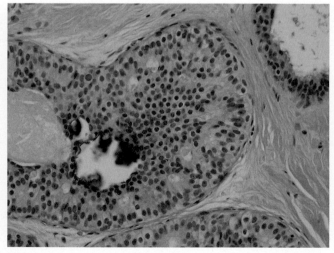

Figure 2.1.9   The uniform cells of ADH form small microrosettes. Cell borders are evident.

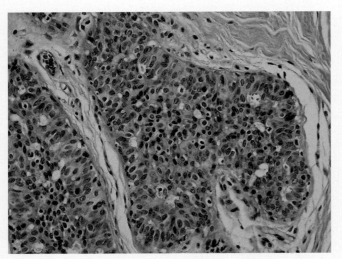

Figure 2.1.5   Fewer secondary spaces are present in this solid, compact focus of florid hyperplasia without atypia, recognized by nuclear variability and overlap.

	Compact Florid Hyperplasia	Solid-Pattern ADH
Age	Adult women	Adult women
Imaging findings	Calcifications or incidental finding	Calcifications or incidental finding
Etiology	Unknown	Unknown
Histology	1. Expansion of terminal duct lobular unit (*Fig. 2.2.1*) 2. Solid growth pattern with few residual secondary lumens (*Figs. 2.2.2–2.2.4*) 3. Nuclear variability (*Figs. 2.2.3 and 2.2.4*) 4. Jumbled cellular arrangement with nuclear overlap, indistinct cell borders, and few, if any, secondary spaces (*Figs. 2.2.3 and 2.2.4*)	1. Affects terminal duct lobular unit (*Fig. 2.2.5*) 2. Solid proliferation of uniform cells partially occupying the involved spaces (*Figs. 2.2.5–2.2.8*) 3. Cells are evenly placed and have distinct cell borders (*Figs. 2.2.7 and 2.2.8*)
Special studies	None; CK5/6 may be expressed in a patchy distribution	None; CK5/6 is usually not expressed
Genetic abnormalities	None	Loss of 16q, 17p
Treatment	Excision not required if detected in a core biopsy specimen	Excision if detected in core biopsy specimen; mammographic follow-up ± antiestrogen therapy
Clinical implication	Slightly increased risk of later cancer development (1.5×); risk level insufficient to affect patient management	Moderately increased risk of later cancer development (4–5×); risk is bilateral

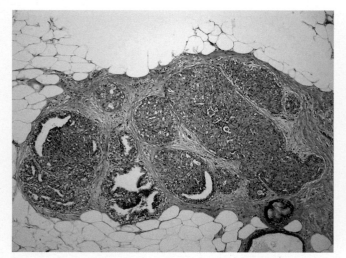

Figure 2.2.1 Florid "compact" pattern hyperplasia without atypia. A lobular unit is expanded and distorted by an epithelial proliferation. A few spaces have residual lumens, but other areas show a solid proliferation without secondary spaces.

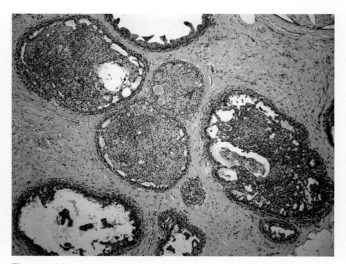

Figure 2.2.5 A lobular unit is expanded by epithelial proliferation.

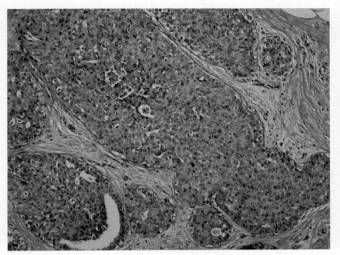

Figure 2.2.2 The epithelial proliferation is exuberant, but indistinct cell borders and nuclear overlap are characteristic of florid hyperplasia without atypia.

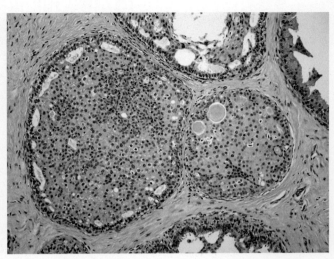

Figure 2.2.6 In this example of ADH, a uniform cell population is interspersed among haphazardly placed cells with overlapping nuclei.

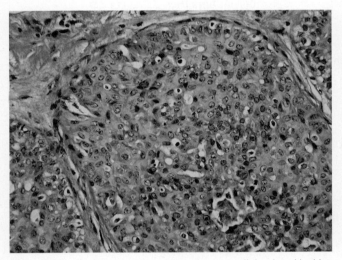

Figure 2.2.3 Nuclear variability and overlap are well developed in this example of florid hyperplasia without atypia.

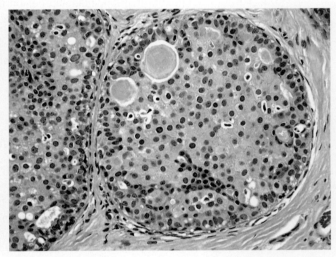

Figure 2.2.7 Cellular monotony and even cell placement characterize the cell population in the central portion of this expanded acinus.

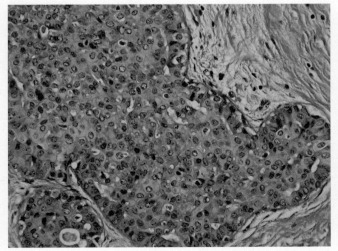

Figure 2.2.4 Occasional "helioid bodies" (apparent nuclear inclusions) are a common feature of florid hyperplasia without atypia. Note the uneven cell placement.

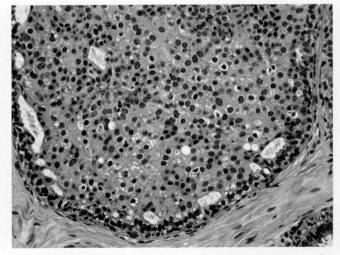

Figure 2.2.8 An important clue to recognizing ADH is the discrete cell borders. Confirmation of partial involvement of acini is the peripheral slit-like spaces and nuclear variability characterizing the cells bordering the basement membrane.

	Florid Hyperplasia Resembling Gynecomastia	Micropapillary-Pattern ADH
Age	Adult women	Adult women
Imaging findings	Calcifications or incidental finding	Calcifications or incidental finding
Etiology	Unknown	Unknown
Histology	1. Cellular proliferation affecting terminal ducts and several lobular units *(Fig. 2.3.1)* 2. Proliferation within terminal duct lobular unit with formation of micropapillae *(Figs. 2.3.2–2.3.5)* 3. Tapering micropapillary projections are composed of cells with pyknotic nuclei; micropapillae appear "stuck on" luminal layer *(Figs. 2.3.3–2.3.5)*	1. Expanded terminal duct lobular unit *(Fig. 2.3.6)* 2. Bulbous micropapillary projections composed of evenly placed, uniform cells *(Figs. 2.3.7 and 2.3.8)* 3. Micropapillae extend from the basement membrane and lack fibrovascular cores *(Figs. 2.3.7 and 2.3.8)*
Special studies	None; there may be patchy expression of CK5/6	None; CK5/6 is usually not expressed
Genetic abnormalities	None	Loss of 16q, 17p
Treatment	No excision necessary if detected in core biopsy specimen	Excision if detected in core biopsy specimen; mammographic follow-up ± antiestrogen therapy
Clinical implication	Slightly increased risk of later cancer development (1.5×); level of risk insufficient to affect patient management	Moderately increased risk of later cancer development (4–5×); risk is bilateral

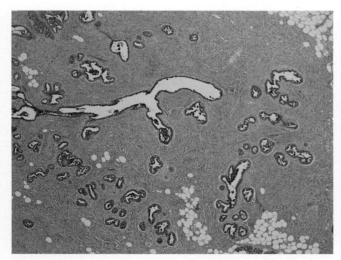

Figure 2.3.1 A terminal duct and surrounding lobular units contain an epithelial proliferation. Note the replacement of loose specialized connective tissue of the lobular unit by fibrous stroma.

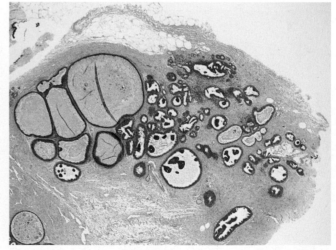

Figure 2.3.6 Micropapillary pattern of ADH. An expanded lobular unit contains rigid micropapillary projections.

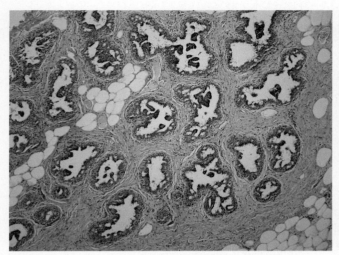

Figure 2.3.2   The acini of this lobular unit have micropapillary projections, some of which bridge the lumen to form an irregular arch.

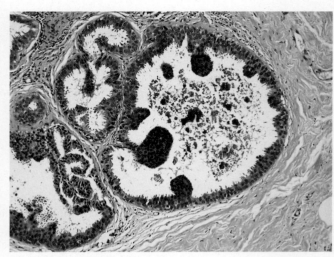

Figure 2.3.7   The micropapillae are bulbous in this example of micropapillary ADH.

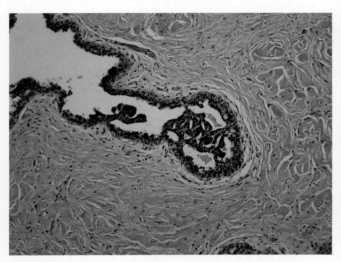

Figure 2.3.3   The stroma surrounding the epithelial proliferation resembles pseudoangiomatous stromal hyperplasia.

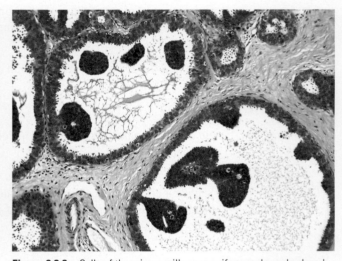

Figure 2.3.8   Cells of the micropapillae are uniform and evenly placed. The micropapillae are rigid and attached to the basement membrane.

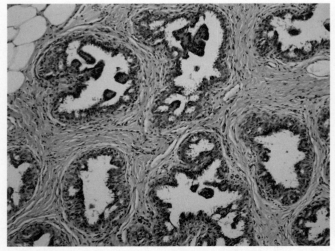

Figure 2.3.4   Cellular bars are nonrigid; micropapillary projections are tapering, and are attached to the luminal layer, which are features of florid hyperplasia without atypia resembling patterns seen in gynecomastia.

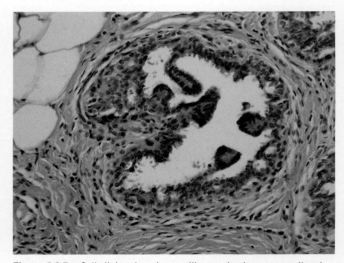

Figure 2.3.5   Cells lining the micropapillary projections are small and pyknotic. The micropapillae have a central clearing in this example of florid hyperplasia without atypia.

	Complex Papillary Apocrine Change	Micropapillary ADH with Apocrine Cytology
Age	Adult women, often perimenopausal	Adult women, usually 55 y or older
Imaging Findings	Calcifications; when present in clustered cysts, may appear as a cystic and solid mass, often incidental	Calcifications
Etiology	Unknown	Unknown
Histology	1. Dilated terminal duct lobular unit lined by apocrine cells *(Figs. 2.4.1 and 2.4.2)* 2. Micropapillary projections lined by apocrine cells extend into lumens *(Figs. 2.4.1–2.4.3)* 3. Fibrovascular cores lined by apocrine cells *(Fig. 2.4.4)* 4. Apocrine cells are bland and contain red apical granules *(Figs. 2.4.4 and 2.4.5)* 5. Micropapillae are delicate, without rigid structure *(Fig. 2.4.5)*	1. Terminal duct lobular unit is expanded and contains numerous micropapillary projections *(Figs. 2.4.6–2.4.8)* 2. Micropapillae are bulbous and lined by uniform cells; fibrovascular cores are lacking *(Figs. 2.4.7 and 2.4.8)* 3. Micropapillae extend into the lumen from the basement membrane, and are composed of cells that are identical to cells that line the acinus *(Fig. 2.4.8)*
Special Studies	None	None; epithelial proliferation usually lacks CK5/6 expression
Genetic abnormalities	None	Loss of 16q, 17p
Treatment	Excision unnecessary	Excision if detected in core biopsy specimen; mammographic follow-up ± antiestrogen therapy
Clinical implication	None	Moderately increased risk of later cancer development (4–5×); risk is bilateral

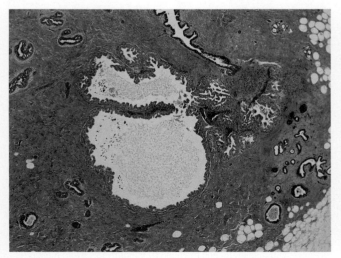

Figure 2.4.1 Papillary apocrine change involving a dilated lobular unit.

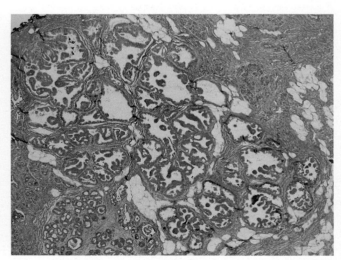

Figure 2.4.6 Uniform cells and bulbous micropapillae partially populate several acini in this example of micropapillary ADH.

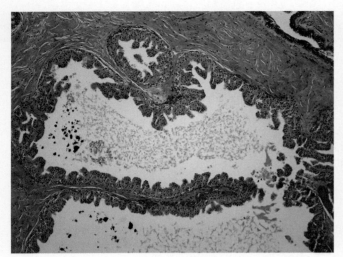

Figure 2.4.2   The apocrine cells that line these spaces form small micropapillary projections along a fibrovascular core.

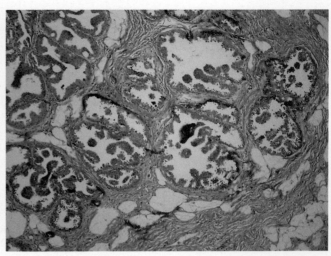

Figure 2.4.7   The bulbous papillae are tethered to the basement membrane rather than appearing "stuck" on the epithelial surface.

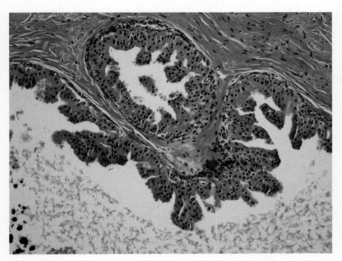

Figure 2.4.3   The apocrine cells are arranged in delicate micropapillae that cross the involved space.

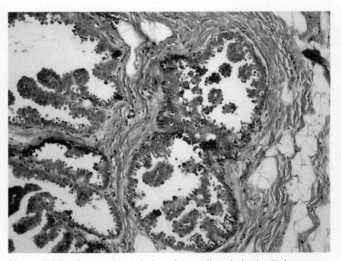

Figure 2.4.8   A second population of normally polarized cells is present between some bulbous papillae.

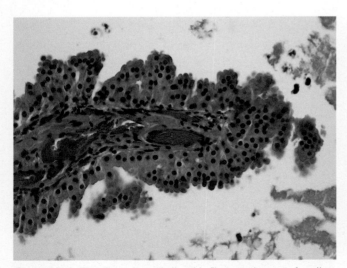

Figure 2.4.4   Bland apocrine cells line this fibrovascular core of papillary apocrine change.

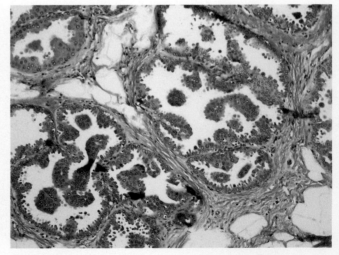

Figure 2.4.5   In ADH the bulbous papillae extend into the lumen from the basement membrane and are lined by uniform cells. Note the lack of fibrovascular cores.

	Cribriform-Pattern ADH	**Collagenous Spherulosis**
Age	Adult women	Adult women
Imaging Findings	Incidental, may be associated with calcification	Incidental finding
Etiology	Unknown	Unknown
Histology	1. Terminal duct lobular unit is expanded by epithelial proliferation *(Figs. 2.5.1 and 2.5.2)* 2. Even cell placement results in rigid secondary spaces *(Figs. 2.5.2–2.5.7)* 3. Cells are uniform and form microrosettes *(Fig. 2.5.6)* 4. Rigid secondary spaces are formed from cells that are arranged perpendicular (not parallel) to the bars and arches *(Fig. 2.5.7)*	1. Round spherules composed of basement membrane material mimic cribriform spaces *(Figs. 2.5.8 and 2.5.9)* 2. Tendrils of epithelium lacking nuclei predominate; nuclei that are present are arranged parallel to the rim of the spherules *(Figs. 2.5.8 and 2.5.9)* 3. Luminal epithelial cells border true lumens *(Fig. 2.5.9)* 4. True lumens contain neutral mucin (blue staining on Alcian Blue/Periodic acid–Schiff [PAS] stain); false lumens contain acidic mucin (pink staining on Alcian Blue/PAS stain), reflective of basement membrane material
Special Studies	None; epithelial proliferation usually lacks CK5/6 expression	Alcian Blue/PAS or immunohistochemistry to detect basement membrane material
Genetic abnormalities	Loss of 16q, 17p	None
Treatment	Excision if detected in core biopsy specimen, mammographic follow-up ± antiestrogen therapy	None
Clinical implication	Moderately increased (bilateral) risk of later cancer development (4–5×)	None

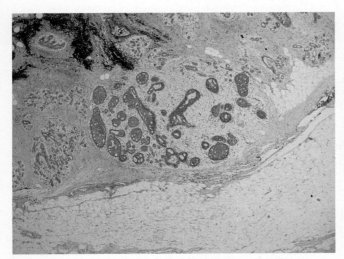

Figure 2.5.1   A lobular unit and part of a terminal duct are expanded by an epithelial proliferation.

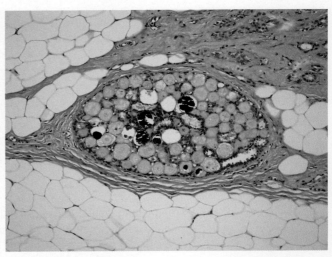

Figure 2.5.8   Collagenous spherulosis: Low-power image suggests cribriform architecture.

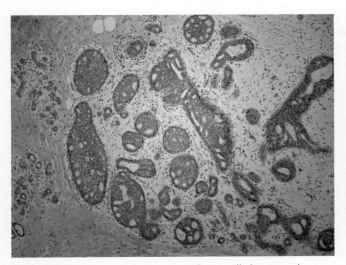

Figure 2.5.2   Rigid secondary spaces and even cell placement characterize this example of ADH.

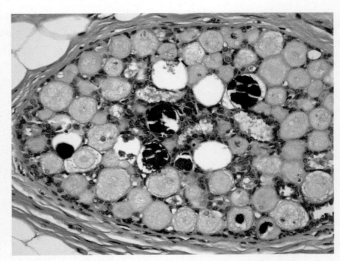

Figure 2.5.9   Spherules containing basement membrane material are responsible for the cribriform architecture in this example of collagenous spherulosis. Note calcifications within the false lumens. Rare true lumens, lined by luminal epithelial cells, are present.

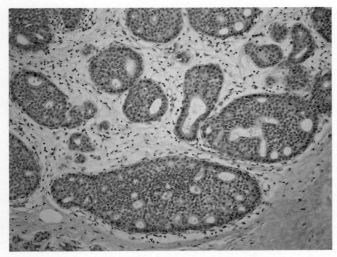

Figure 2.5.3   In ADH the cell borders are distinct, and even cell placement results in crisp secondary spaces.

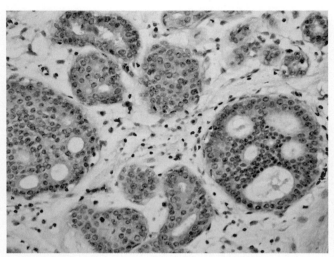

Figure 2.5.4   The bars and arches of ADH are composed of uniform bland cells.

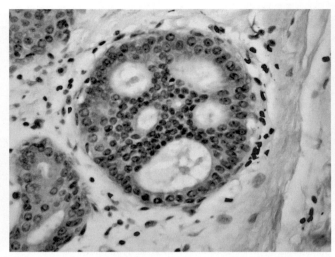

Figure 2.5.7   Incomplete involvement of this space by cellular uniformity qualifies as ADH. Some cellular bars are thickened and uniform, while the cribriform space in the upper right is composed predominantly of cytoplasm.

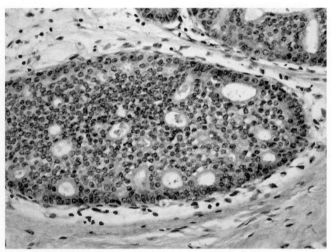

Figure 2.5.5   Some secondary spaces are irregular, but other cribriform structures are sharply defined by evenly arranged uniform cells in this example of ADH.

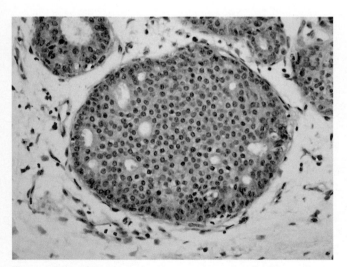

Figure 2.5.6   ADH characterized by even placement of uniform cells.

SUGGESTED READINGS

Collins Lc, Baer Hj, Tamimi Rm, Et Al. Magnitude And Laterality Of Breast Cancer Risk According To Histologic Type Of Atypical Hyperplasia: Results From The Nurses' Health Study. *Cancer.* 2007;109:180–187.

Dupont Wd, Page Dl. Risk Factors For Breast Cancer In Women With Proliferative Breast Disease. *N Engl J Med.* 1985;312:146–151.

Dupont Wd, Page Dl. Relative Risk Cf Breast Cancer Varies With Time Since Diagnosis Of Atypical Hyperplasia. *Hum Pathol.* 1989;20:723-5.

Hartmann Lc, Sellers Ta, Frost Mh, Et Al. Benign Breast Disease And The Risk Of Breast Cancer. *N Engl J Med.* 2005;353:229–237.

Jensen Ra, Page Dl. Epithelial Hyperpasia. In: Elston Cw, Ellis Io, Eds. *The Breast.* 3Rd Ed. Edinburgh: Churchill Livingstone; 1988:65–89.

Kelsey Jl, Gammon Md, John Em. Reproductive Factors And Breast Cancer. *Epidemiol Rev.* 1993;15:36–47.

London Sj, Connolly Jl, Schnitt Sj, Et Al. A Prospective Study Of Benign Breast Disease And The Risk Of Breast Cancer. *Jama.* 1992;267:941–944.

Marshall Lm, Hunter Dj, Connolly Jl, Et Al. Risk Of Breast Cancer Associated With Atypical Hyperplasia Of Lobular And Ductal Types. *Cancer Epidemiol Biomarkers Prev.* 1997;6:297–301.

Page Dl, Dupont Wd, Jensen Ra. Papillary Apocrine Change Of The Breast: Associations With Atypical Hyperplasia And Risk Of Breast Cancer. *Cancer Epidemiol Biomarkers Prev.* 1996;5:29–32.

Page Dl, Dupont Wd, Rogers Lw, Et Al. Atypical Hyperplastic Lesions Of The Female Breast: A Long-Term Follow-Up Study. *Cancer.* 1985;55:2698–2708.

Tavassoli Fa, Norris Hj. A Comparison Of The Results Of Long-Term Follow-Up For Atypical Intraductal Hyperplasia And Intraductal Hyperplasia Of The Breast. *Cancer.* 1990;65:518–529.

3

Lobular Neoplasia and Its Distinction from Other Epithelial Proliferative Lesions

	Florid Hyperplasia with Clear Cells	Atypical Lobular Hyperplasia (ALH)
Age	Adult women	Adult women, incidence drops following menopause
Imaging findings	Incidental finding or associated with calcifications	Incidental finding, rarely associated with calcifications
Etiology	Unknown	Unknown
Histology	1. Lobular unit expanded by a proliferation of nonuniform epithelial cells with residual secondary lumens *(Fig. 3.1.1)* 2. Secondary spaces are irregular, with a slit-like arrangement *(Figs. 3.1.2–3.1.4)* 3. Nuclear variability and overlap are evident *(Figs. 3.1.2–3.1.4)* 4. Indistinct cell borders *(Figs. 3.1.3 and 3.1.4)*	1. Lobular units contain a uniform cell population, with some filling of acini by small cells with a dyshesive growth pattern *(Figs. 3.1.5 and 3.1.6)* 2. Acini contain characteristic cells, but are not fully distended, and are not distorted *(Figs. 3.1.5–3.1.8)* 3. Residual luminal epithelial and myoepithelial cells are present *(Figs. 3.1.7 and 3.1.8)* 4. Intracytoplasmic inclusions are common *(Fig. 3.1.8)*
Special studies	None; CK5/6 may be variably expressed	None; E-cadherin is usually not expressed; p120 expression maintained
Genetic abnormalities	None	Mutations of *CDH1* (chromosome 16q22.1)
Treatment	None	Excision not required if incidental finding on core biopsy; mammographic follow-up ± anti-estrogen therapy
Clinical implication	Slightly increased risk of later cancer development (1.5×); magnitude of risk insufficient to affect patient management	Moderately increased risk of later cancer development (4–5×); bilateral risk with ipsilateral breast at greater (3:1) risk

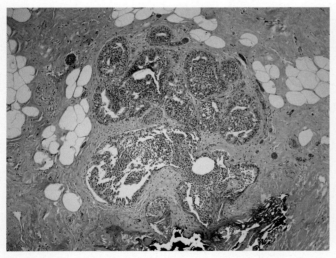

Figure 3.1.1   A lobular unit is expanded by an epithelial proliferation with irregular secondary spaces characteristic of florid hyperplasia.

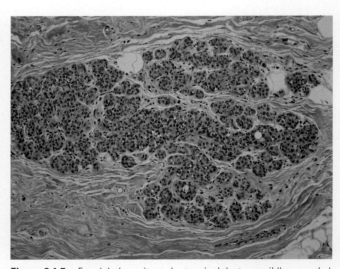

Figure 3.1.5   Four lobular units and a terminal duct are mildly expanded by a uniform population of cells in this example of ALH.

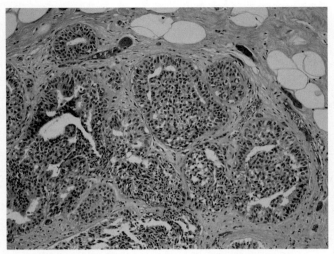

Figure 3.1.2   Uneven cell placement and peripheral slit-like spaces define florid hyperplasia without atypia; cells are polarized with respect to the basement membrane.

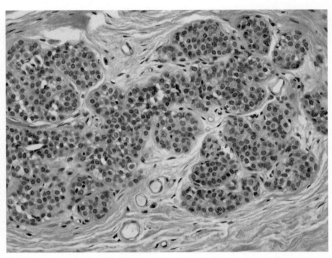

Figure 3.1.6   The acini contain a uniform population of cells that are evenly placed. A dyshesive growth pattern is evident, as well as a few residual lumina in some acini. The involved spaces are minimally expanded, and there is no distortion.

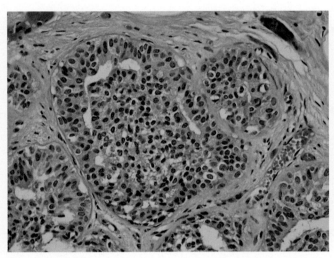

Figure 3.1.3   Many of the epithelial cells have clear cytoplasm which may suggest cellular monotony.

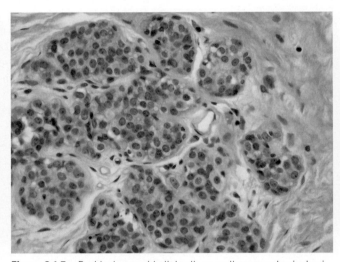

Figure 3.1.7   Residual myoepithelial cells as well as some luminal epithelial cells remain which are admixed with ALH cells.

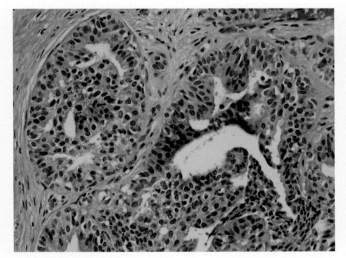

Figure 3.1.4   Indistinct cell borders, nuclear variability, and uneven cell placement are features of florid hyperplasia without atypia.

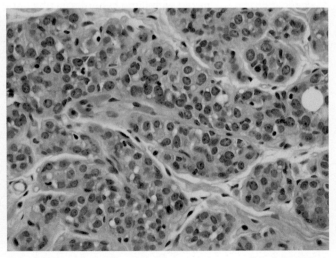

Figure 3.1.8   Many of the ALH cells contain intracytoplasmic inclusions.

3 Lobular Neoplasia

	Usual Hyperplasia with Prominent Myoepithelial Cells	ALH
Age	Adult women	Adult women, incidence drops following menopause
Imaging findings	Incidental finding, or associated with calcifications	Incidental finding, rarely associated with calcifications
Etiology	Unknown	Unknown
Histology	1. Nonuniform cellular proliferation involving clustered lobular units *(Fig. 3.2.1)* 2. Mixture of cell types; myoepithelial cells are recognized by clear cytoplasm and peripheral location while central luminal epithelial cells have eosinophilic cytoplasm *(Figs. 3.2.1–3.2.4)* 3. Nuclear variability and overlap are present in both cell populations *(Figs. 3.2.2–3.2.4)* 4. Irregular secondary spaces and myoepithelial cells with clear cytoplasm *(Figs. 3.2.2–3.2.4)* 5. Myoepithelial cells lack intracytoplasmic inclusions *(Figs. 3.2.2–3.2.4)*	1. Lobular units are variably populated by uniform cells with a dyshesive growth pattern *(Figs. 3.2.5 and 3.2.6)* 2. Evenly placed, uniform cells lack well-defined cellular borders, and acini are not filled or distended *(Figs. 3.2.6–3.2.8)* 3. Intracytoplasmic inclusions are frequent *(Fig. 3.2.8)* 4. Acini are closely opposed, but intervening stroma is evident *(Fig. 3.2.8)*
Special studies	None; CK5/6, and E-cadherin diffusely expressed	None; E-cadherin is usually not expressed, intact p120 expression
Genetic abnormalities	None	Mutations of *CDH1* (chromosome 16q22.1)
Treatment	Excision unnecessary if detected in core biopsy specimen	Excision not required if incidental finding on core biopsy; mammographic follow-up ± antiestrogen therapy
Clinical implication	Risk implications apply only when present admixed with florid hyperplasia, the latter being the risk-indicator lesion; slightly increased risk of later cancer development (1.5×); risk is bilateral. Risk level is insufficient to affect patient management.	Moderately increased risk of later cancer development (4–5×); bilateral risk with ipsilateral breast at greater (3:1) risk

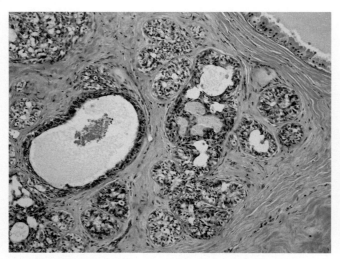

Figure 3.2.1   Acini are minimally expanded by cells with clear cytoplasm. Some acini contain irregular secondary spaces.

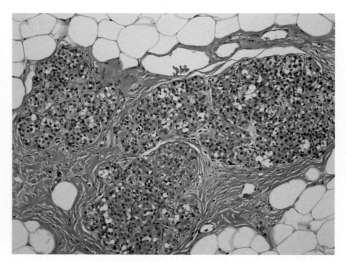

Figure 3.2.5   Four lobular units are mildly expanded by a proliferation of cells in this example of ALH. The cellular uniformity is evident at low power.

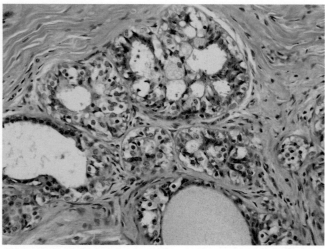

Figure 3.2.2   The periphery of the acini contain a proliferation of myoepithelial cells with characteristic clear cytoplasm. Luminal epithelial cells with eosinophilic cytoplasm line the secondary spaces. Note uneven cell placement in both populations.

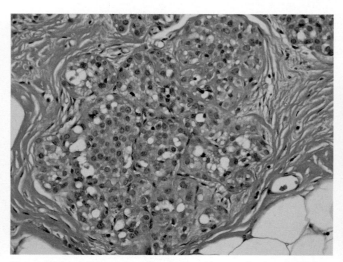

Figure 3.2.6   Acini contain uniform cells with centrally placed nuclei. The dyshesive nature of the cells is evident.

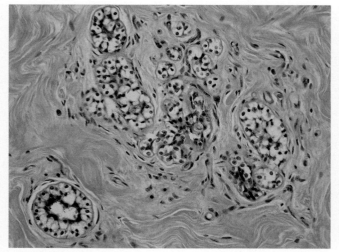

Figure 3.2.3   This atrophic lobular unit is composed almost exclusively of myoepithelial cells with clear cytoplasm, with scant residual luminal epithelial cells present centrally.

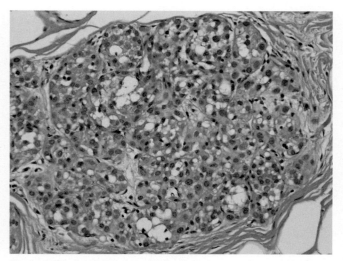

Figure 3.2.7   In this lobular unit, the dyshesive growth pattern is more pronounced. Numerous intracytoplasmic inclusions are evident and multiple acini have residual intercellular lumens.

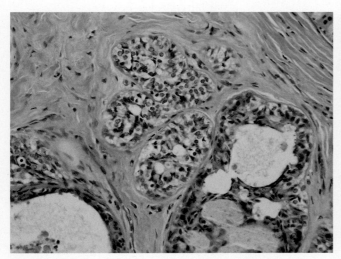

Figure 3.2.4 Acini mildly expanded by myoepithelial cells with clear cytoplasm and rare interspersed luminal epithelial cells are adjacent to a space showing usual hyperplasia and peripheral myoepithlial cells.

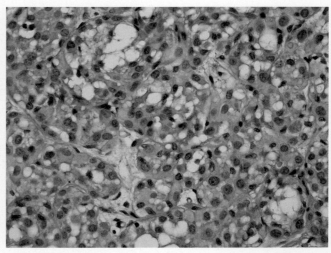

Figure 3.2.8 Many of the cells of ALH have intracytoplasmic inclusions. Admixed residual luminal epithelial cells are evident, characterized by dark, attenuated nuclei.

	ALH	Solid-Pattern Atypical Ductal Hyperplasia (ADH)
Age	Adult women, incidence drops following menopause	Adult women
Imaging findings	Incidental finding, rarely associated with calcifications	Calcifications or incidental finding
Etiology	Unknown	Unknown
Histology	1. Lobular units are expanded by a cellular proliferation with a solid growth pattern *(Figs. 3.3.1 and 3.3.2)* 2. Cellular uniformity and dyshesion are evident at low power *(Figs. 3.3.3 and 3.3.4)* 3. Acini are filled by small uniform cells, with scant space remaining between cells (an important differential point for lobular carcinoma in situ [LCIS]; see Section 3.4) *(Fig. 3.3.3)* 4. Acini may be partially involved, with residual intercellular lumina *(Fig. 3.3.4)* 5. Intracytoplasmic inclusions are common *(Fig. 3.3.4)*	1. Terminal duct lobular unit shows expansion by a cellular proliferation *(Fig. 3.3.5)* 2. Acini contain a central, solid proliferation of uniform cells *(Figs. 3.3.6 and 3.3.7)* 3. Cells have uniform nuclei and are evenly placed with distinct cell borders; occasional microrosettes are present *(Fig. 3.3.7)*
Special studies	None; E-cadherin is usually not expressed	None; CK5/6 usually not expressed
Genetic abnormalities	Mutations of *CDH1* (chromosome 16q22.1); p120 expression maintained	Loss of 16q, 17p
Treatment	Excision not required if incidental finding on core biopsy; mammographic follow-up ± antiestrogen therapy	Excision if detected in core biopsy specimen; mammographic follow-up ± antiestrogen therapy.
Clinical implication	Moderately increased risk of later cancer development (4–5×); bilateral risk with ipsilateral breast at greater (3:1) risk	Moderately increased risk of later cancer development (4–5×); risk is bilateral

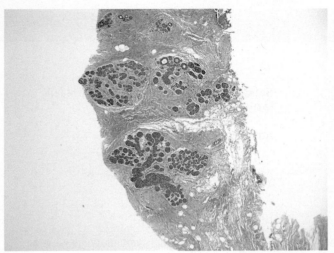

Figure 3.3.1 This core biopsy specimen contains several lobular units expanded by a cellular proliferation.

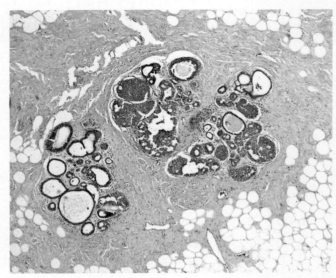

Figure 3.3.5 ADH, solid pattern: Two adjacent lobular units are partially involved by a solid epithelial proliferation (*center*).

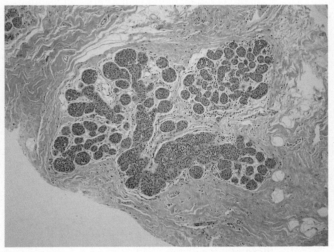

Figure 3.3.2 The cellular uniformity and even cell placement of ALH are evident at low power.

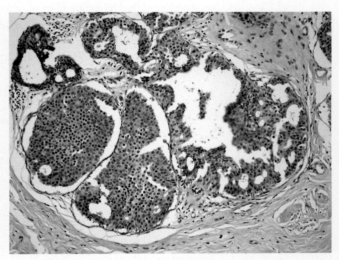

Figure 3.3.6 Cellular uniformity and even cell placement are evident in solid-pattern ADH.

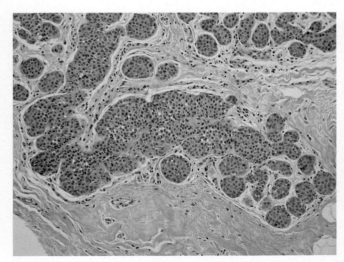

Figure 3.3.3 A dyshesive growth pattern characterizes ALH. Variable involvement of terminal ducts is a frequent feature and does not equate with LCIS.

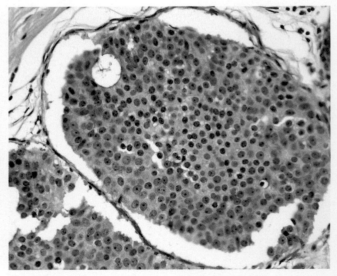

Figure 3.3.7 Distinct cell borders and the presence of occasional microrosettes are characteristic of solid-pattern ADH. The cells are cohesive.

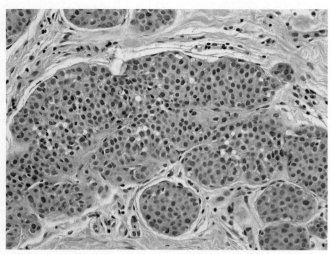

Figure 3.3.4   Discrete, cohesive intercellular borders are not a feature of ALH, rather, cells are dyshesive. Scattered intracytoplasmic inclusions are present.

	ALH	LCIS
Age	Adult women, incidence drops following menopause	Adult women, incidence drops following menopause
Imaging findings	Incidental finding, rarely associated with calcifications	Incidental finding, rarely associated with calcifications
Etiology	Unknown	Unknown
Histology	1. Lobular units are mildly expanded by a cellular proliferation with a solid growth pattern *(Figs. 3.4.1–3.4.3)* 2. Cellular uniformity and a dyshesive growth pattern are evident at low power *(Fig. 3.4.1)* 3. Acini are filled by small uniform cells, with scant space remaining between cells *(Fig. 3.4.3)* 4. Intracytoplasmic inclusions are common *(Fig. 3.4.3)*	1. More than half of the acini of this lobular unit are markedly distended and distorted by a cellular proliferation *(Figs. 3.4.4 and 3.4.5)* 2. Uniform cells are evenly placed with a dyshesive growth pattern, often with intra-cytoplasmic inclusions *(Figs. 3.4.6 and 3.4.7)* 3. Characteristic cells often show pagetoid growth along ducts *(Fig. 3.4.5)*
Special studies	None to distinguish from LCIS; E-cadherin is usually not expressed, p120 expression maintained	None to distinguish from ALH; E-cadherin is usually not expressed *(Fig. 3.4.8)*; p120 expression maintained
Genetic abnormalities	Mutations of *CDH1* (chromosome 16q22.1)	Mutations of *CDH1* (chromosome 16q22.1)
Treatment	Excision not required if incidental finding on core biopsy; mammographic follow-up ± anti-estrogen therapy	Excision not required if incidental finding in core biopsy specimen; mammographic follow-up ± antiestrogen therapy
Clinical implication	Moderately increased risk of later cancer development (4–5×); bilateral risk with ipsilateral breast at greater (3:1) risk	High relative risk (9–10×) of later cancer development; bilateral risk with ipsilateral breast at greater (3:1) risk; risk drops following menopause

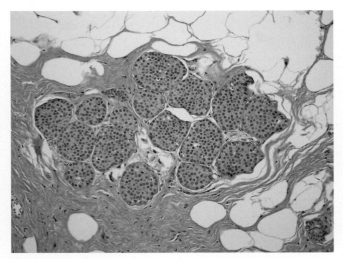

Figure 3.4.1   ALH: The acini of this lobular unit contain a proliferation of characteristic cells; however, marked distention and distortion of the involved spaces are lacking.

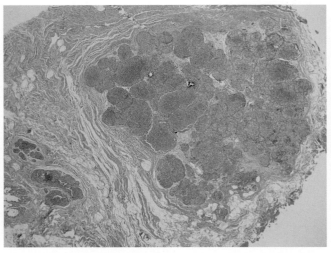

Figure 3.4.4   Marked distention and distortion of the involved spaces defines LCIS (right). Pagetoid spread along ducts (left) is frequent.

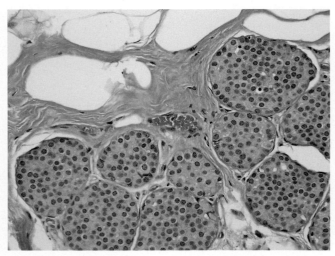

Figure 3.4.2   The degree of cellular proliferation qualifies as ALH, because half of the acini lack distortion.

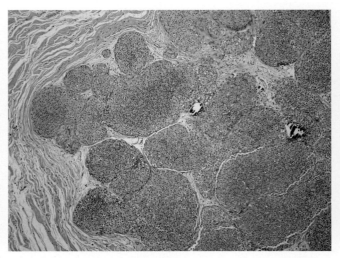

Figure 3.4.5   Small uniform cells have a dyshesive growth pattern. The cell type is identical to ALH; however, LCIS is diagnosed because of the marked distention and distortion of more than half of the involved spaces.

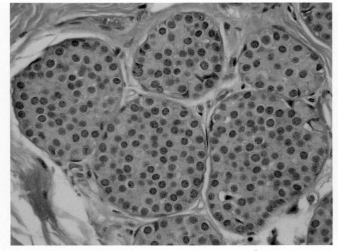

Figure 3.4.3   The two acini at the top have only five or six cells across, qualifying as ALH.

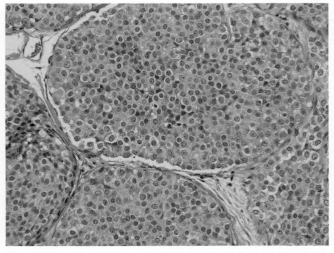

Figure 3.4.6   All acini are markedly distended and distorted. No normal luminal epithelial cells remain.

3 Lobular Neoplasia

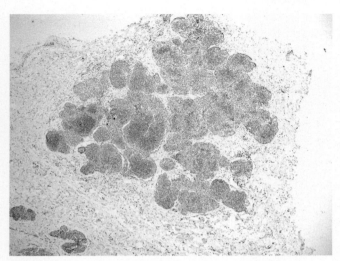

Figure 3.4.7   E-cadherin expression is absent in this example of LCIS.

	LCIS	Compact Florid Hyperplasia without Atypia
Age	Adult women, incidence drops following menopause	Adult women
Imaging findings	Incidental finding, rarely associated with calcification	Calcifications, incidental finding, or solid nodule
Etiology	Unknown	Unknown
Histology	1. Lobular units are distended and distorted by a cellular proliferation *(Figs. 3.5.1–3.5.3)* 2. Uniform cells are evenly placed with a dyshesive growth pattern, often with intra-cytoplasmic inclusions *(Figs. 3.5.3–3.5.5)* 3. Characteristic cells often show pagetoid growth along ducts *(Fig. 3.5.2)*	1. Terminal duct lobular unit is expanded by a proliferation of epithelial cells *(Fig. 3.5.7)* 2. Solid growth pattern without secondary spaces *(Figs. 3.5.8–3.5.10)* 3. Cells are unevenly placed, with indistinct cell borders *(Figs. 3.5.8–3.5.10)* 4. Nuclear variability and overlap *(Figs. 3.5.8–3.5.10)*; cells are arranged in a swirling or streaming pattern *(Figs. 3.5.8–3.5.10)*
Special studies	None; E-cadherin is usually not expressed *(Fig. 3.5.6)*; p120 expression present	None; CK 5/6 is variably expressed
Genetic abnormalities	Mutations of *CDH1* (chromosome 16q22.1)	None
Treatment	Excision not required if incidental finding in core biopsy specimen; mammographic follow-up ± antiestrogen therapy	Excision not required
Clinical implication	High relative risk (9–10×) of later cancer development; bilateral risk with ipsilateral breast at greater (3:1) risk; risk drops following menopause	Slightly increased risk of later cancer development (1.5×); risk is bilateral. Risk level is insufficient to affect patient management.

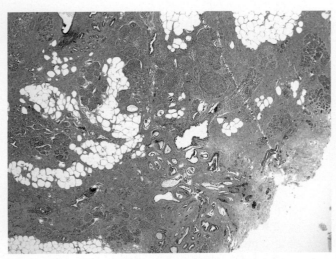

Figure 3.5.1   Several lobular units associated with this radial scar show a marked cellular proliferation.

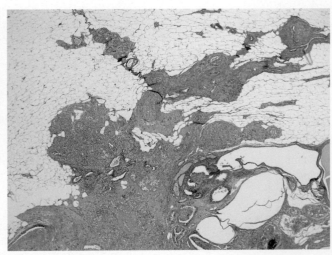

Figure 3.5.7   Several lobular units radiating from this radial scar show a cellular proliferation.

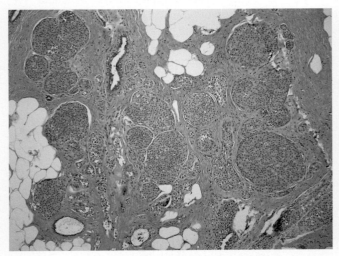

Figure 3.5.2   More than half of the acini of the lobular units are distended and distorted by the proliferation. A terminal duct (upper left) shows pagetoid spread of lobular neoplasia cells.

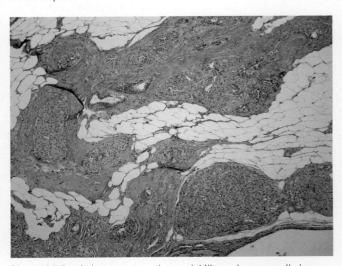

Figure 3.5.8   At low power, nuclear variability and uneven cell placement create a "swirling" pattern in this example of florid hyperplasia without atypia.

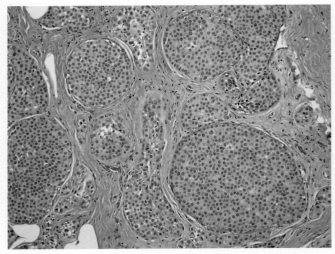

Figure 3.5.3   Despite the distention and distortion, the proliferation involves lobular units, not true ducts. Uniform, evenly placed, dyshesive cells characterize LCIS.

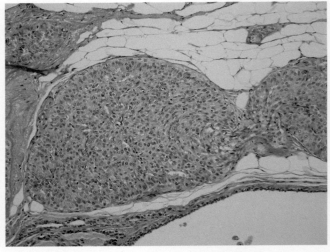

Figure 3.5.9   In compact or solid-pattern florid hyperplasia without atypia, nuclear overlap and uneven cell placement are defining.

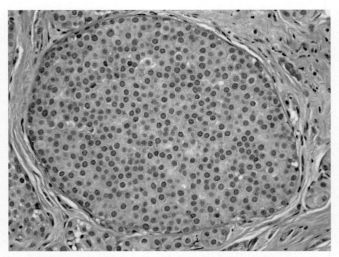

Figure 3.5.4   LCIS: Uniform cells have a dyshesive growth pattern.

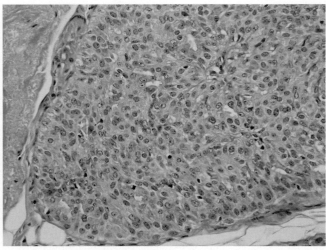

Figure 3.5.10   The cells are jumbled, with nuclear overlap and variability. The cell borders are indistinct, characteristic of florid hyperplasia without atypia.

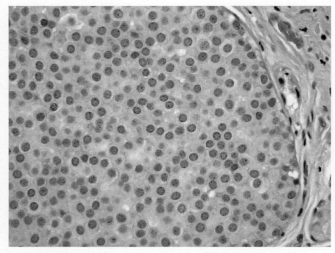

Figure 3.5.5   Small bland, centrally placed nuclei are characteristic of both ALH and LCIS. The distinction is based on the degree of distention and distortion, well-illustrated in this example of LCIS

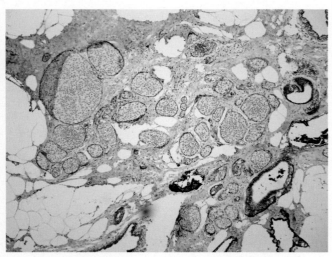

Figure 3.5.6   E-Cadherin immunohistochemical study. LCIS is almost uniformly negative for expression of this cell adhesion molecule.

3 Lobular Neoplasia

SUGGESTED READINGS

Acs G, Lawton TJ, Rebbeck TR, et al. Differential expression of E-cadherin in lobular and ductal neoplasms of the breast and its biologic and diagnostic implications. *Am J Clin Pathol.* 2001;115:85–98.

Anderson JA. Lobular carcinoma in situ. A histological study of 52 cases. *Acta Pathol Microbiol Scand A.* 1974;82:735–741.

Carter BA, Page DL, Schuyler P, et al. No elevation in long-term breast carcinoma risk for women with fibroadenomas that contain atypical hyperplasia. *Cancer.* 2001;92:30–36.

Collins LC. Does the extent of atypical hyperplasia in a benign breast biopsyinfluence the magnitude of breast cancer risk? An update from the Nurses' Health Study. *Mod Pathol.* 2013;26:34A:133.

Collins LC, Baer HJ, Tamimi RM, et al. Magnitude and laterality of breast cancer risk according to histologic type of atypical hyperplasia: results from the Nurses' Health Study. *Cancer.* 2007;109:180–187.

Foote F, Stewart, F. Lobular carcinoma in situ: a rare form of mammary carcinoma. *Am J Pathol.* 1941;17:491–496.

Haagensen CD, Lane N, Lattes R, et al. Lobular neoplasia (so-called lobular carcinoma in situ) of the breast. *Cancer.* 1978;42:737–769.

Hartmann LC, Sellers TA, Frost MH, et al. Benign breast disease and the risk of breast cancer. *N Engl J Med.* 2005;353:229–237.

Marshall LM, Hunter DJ, Connolly JL, et al. Risk of breast cancer associated with atypical hyperplasia of lobular and ductal types. *Cancer Epidemiol Biomarkers Prev.* 1997;6:297–301.

Page DL, Dupont WD, Rogers LW. Ductal involvement by cells of atypical lobular hyperplasia in the breast: a long-term follow-up study of cancer risk. *Hum Pathol.* 1988;19:201–207.

Page DL, Dupont WD, Rogers LW, et al. Atypical hyperplastic lesions of the female breast. A long-term follow-up study. *Cancer.* 1985;55:2698–2708.

Page DL, Kidd TE Jr, Dupont WD, et al. Lobular neoplasia of the breast: higher risk for subsequent invasive cancer predicted by more extensive disease. *Hum Pathol.* 1991;22:1232–1239.

Page DL, Schuyler PA, Dupont WD, et al. Atypical lobular hyperplasia as a unilateral predictor of breast cancer risk: a retrospective cohort study. *Lancet.* 2003;361:125–129.

Rosen PP, Braun DW Jr, Lyngholm B, et al. Lobular carcinoma in situ of the breast: preliminary results of treatment by ipsilateral mastectomy and contralateral breast biopsy. *Cancer.* 1981;47:813–819.

Rosen PP, Kosloff C, Lieberman PH, et al. Lobular carcinoma in situ of the breast. Detailed analysis of 99 patients with average follow-up of 24 years. *Am J Surg Pathol.* 1978;2:225–251.

Wheeler JE, Enterline HT, Roseman JM, et al. Lobular carcinoma in situ of the breast. Long-term followup. *Cancer.* 1974;34:554–563.

4

Ductal Carcinoma In Situ

	Cribriform Atypical Ductal Hyperplasia (ADH)	Low-Grade Ductal Carcinoma In Situ (DCIS)
Age	Adult women	Adult women, usually older than 50 y
Location	Anywhere in the breast	Anywhere in the breast
Imaging findings	Calcifications, or incidental finding	Calcifications, rarely mass-forming
Etiology	Unknown	Unknown
Histology	1. Terminal duct lobular unit contains a uniform proliferation of small, bland cells with distinct cell borders and even cell placement but process incompletely occupies the involved spaces *(Figs. 4.1.1–4.1.5)* 2. Rigid architecture consisting of cribriform spaces or mixed solid and cribriform areas *(Figs. 4.1.2–4.1.4)* 3. Subtle microrosettes may be present *(Fig. 4.1.5)* 4. Limited extent, usually confined to the terminal duct lobular unit and measuring less than 2 mm *(Fig. 4.1.1)*	1. Terminal duct lobular units, as well as true ducts contain a uniform proliferation of small bland cells *(Figs. 4.1.6–4.1.10)* 2. Complete involvement of at least two adjacent spaces, equivalent to a linear extent of at least 3 mm *(Figs. 4.1.6–4.1.8)* 3. Cell borders are distinct, and cells are evenly placed *(Fig. 4.1.9)* 4. Rigid architecture with cribriform or micropapillary patterns most common *(Figs. 4.1.7–4.1.10)*; solid growth pattern may contain microrosettes 5. True duct involvement often *(Figs. 4.1.6 and 4.1.7)*
Special studies	None, CK5/6 usually not expressed	None; CK5/6 usually not expressed; estrogen receptor (ER) routinely assessed to predict response to adjuvant endocrine therapy; multigene assay may predict which patients may be spared radiation
Genetic abnormalities	Loss of 16q, 17p	Loss of 16q, 17p
Treatment	Excision if detected in core biopsy, mammographic follow-up ± antiestrogen therapy	Complete excision with negative margins, ± adjuvant radiation, ± antiestrogen therapy; sentinel lymph node biopsy not indicated
Clinical implication	Moderately increased risk of later cancer development (4–5×); risk is bilateral	Development of invasive carcinoma in approximately 30% of cases if incompletely excised; with complete excision recurrence rate is approximately 5%–8% without radiation; when limited in extent recurrence rate <5%

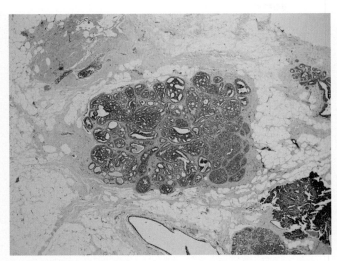

Figure 4.1.1   ADH: A lobular unit is expanded by a proliferation of cells showing rigid architecture.

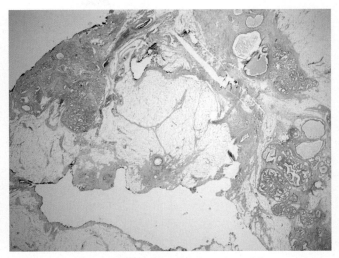

Figure 4.1.6   Low-grade DCIS. Three lobular units and ducts are populated by uniform cells with rigid architecture.

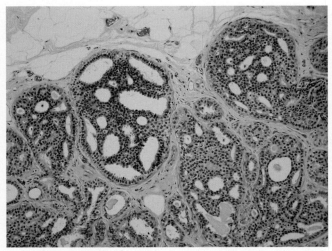

Figure 4.1.2   Several acini are partially populated by monotonous cells in ADH; note residual normally polarized cells at periphery of spaces and occasional irregularly shaped secondary spaces.

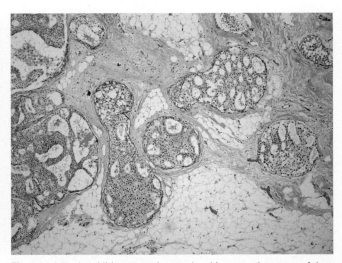

Figure 4.1.7   In addition to cytology and architecture, the extent of the proliferation, including involvement of true ducts, qualifies as DCIS.

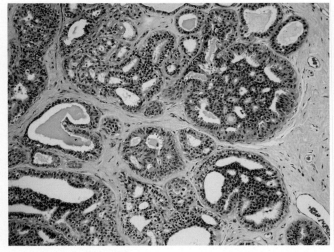

Figure 4.1.3   Uniform, evenly placed cells are present centrally in the involved spaces (right of center), while the cells at the periphery of the acini lack uniformity and maintain normal polarity, qualifying as ADH.

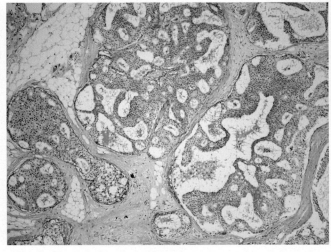

Figure 4.1.8   Secretory material should not be misinterpreted as necrosis in this example of low-grade DCIS.

4 Ductal Carcinoma In Situ

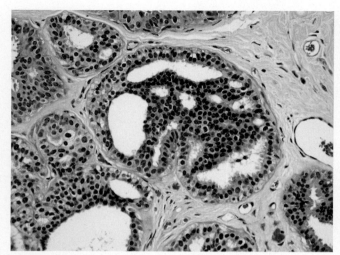

Figure 4.1.4   Despite cellular monotony, the peripheral secondary spaces are irregular in this example of ADH.

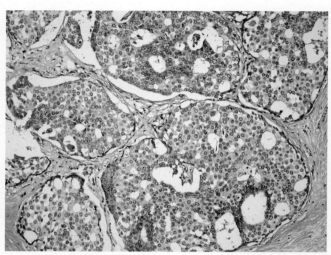

Figure 4.1.9   The involved spaces are contiguous and completely replaced by the atypical cells, underscoring the importance of the extent of involvement in making the determination of DCIS.

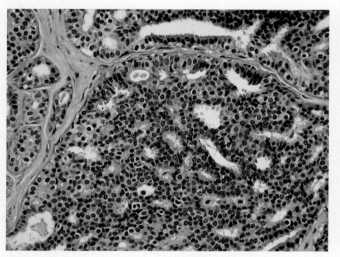

Figure 4.1.5   Uniform cells form microrosettes in this example of ADH.

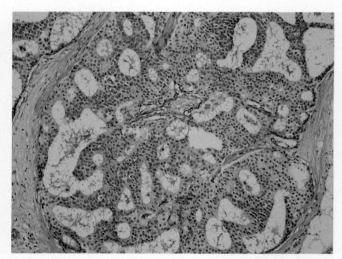

Figure 4.1.10   Low-grade DCIS: Uniform cell population with distinct cell borders forms crisp secondary spaces.

	Micropapillary ADH	**Micropapillary DCIS**
Age	Adult women	Adult women
Location	Anywhere in the breast	Anywhere in the breast
Imaging findings	Calcifications or incidental finding	Calcifications, rarely mass or nipple discharge
Etiology	Unknown	Unknown
Histology	1. Epithelial proliferation limited to partial involvement of the terminal duct lobular unit *(Figs. 4.2.1–4.2.5)* 2. Bulbous micropapillary projections composed of evenly placed, uniform cells *(Figs. 4.2.4 and 4.2.5)*; second population of normally polarized cells remains 3. Micropapillae extend from the basement membrane and lack fibrovascular cores *(Figs. 4.2.4 and 4.2.5)*	1. Micropapillary proliferation involving several expanded lobular units and ducts *(Figs. 4.2.6–4.2.10)* 2. Proliferation of uniform cells evenly placed within bulbous micropapillae *(Figs. 4.2.8–4.2.10)* 3. Micropapillae lack fibrovascular cores and extend into lumen from basement membrane *(Figs. 4.2.8–4.2.10)* 4. May be of low, intermediate, or high nuclear grade, although differential diagnostic partner with ADH is low-grade DCIS *(Fig. 4.2.10)* 5. May be present in a patchy distribution within individual lobular units; however, numerous contiguously involved spaces support a diagnosis of micropapillary DCIS *(Fig. 4.2.6)*
Special studies	None; CK5/6 is usually not expressed	None; CK5/6 usually not expressed; ER expression routinely assessed to predict response to adjuvant endocrine therapy; multigene assay may predict which patients may be spared radiation
Genetic abnormalities	Loss of 16q, 17p	Loss of 16q, 17p
Treatment	Excision if detected in core biopsy specimen; mammographic follow-up, ± antiestrogen therapy	Complete excision with negative margins, ± adjuvant radiation, ± antiestrogen therapy; sentinel lymph node biopsy not indicated. Pure micropapillary DCIS may be extensively present in the breast, requiring mastectomy.
Clinical implication	Moderately increased risk of later cancer development (4–5×); risk is bilateral	Development of invasive carcinoma in approximately 30% of cases if incompletely excised; with complete excision, recurrence rate approximately 5%–8% without radiation; recurrence rate less than 5% for low grade DCIS of limited extent

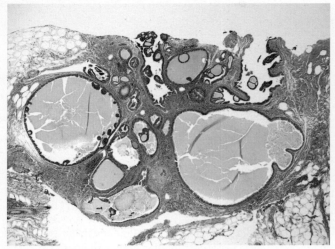

Figure 4.2.1   ADH: A core needle biopsy specimen contains an expanded lobular unit; several of the spaces contain bulbous micropapillary projections.

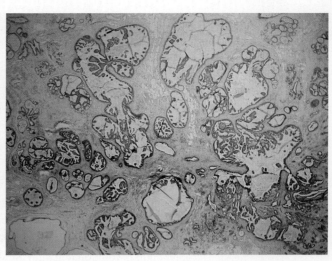

Figure 4.2.6   Micropapillary DCIS (low grade): Several adjacent lobular units and intervening ducts contain a proliferation of micropapillae, with a "shaggy" appearance at low power.

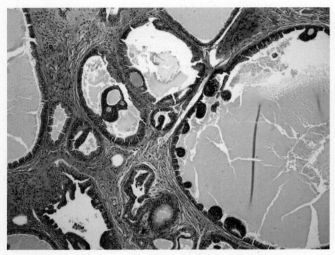

Figure 4.2.2   Cellular uniformity of the micropapillary projections of ADH is evident even on low power.

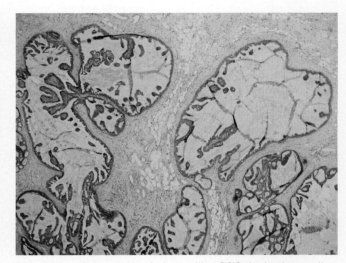

Figure 4.2.7   This example of micropapillary DCIS also involves papillomas, explaining the presence of papillary projections with fibrovascular cores.

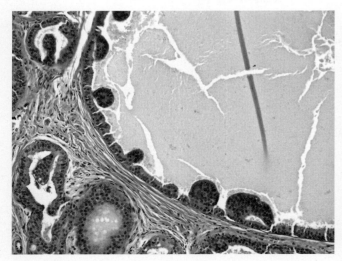

Figure 4.2.3   Normally polarized cells are present between the micropapillae in this example of ADH.

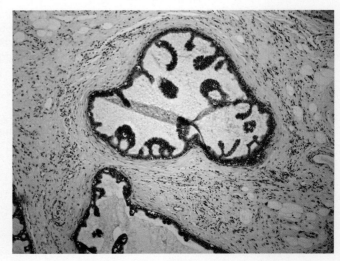

Figure 4.2.8   The micropapillae of DCIS are bulbous, with even cell placement; the architectural complexity of the proliferation is evidenced by the presence of seemingly unattached cell clusters within lumens.

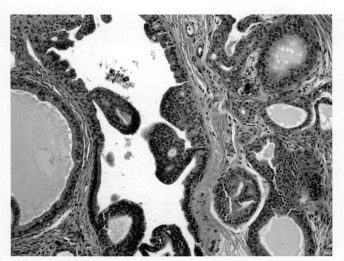

Figure 4.2.4   Micropapillae of ADH lack fibrovascular cores.

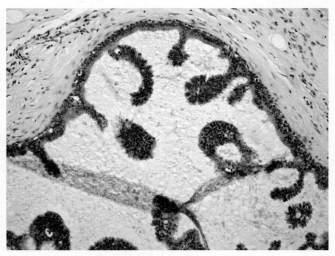

Figure 4.2.9   Cells forming the micropapillae are similar to the adjacent cells lining the expanded spaces in this example of DCIS.

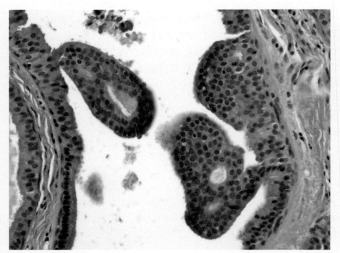

Figure 4.2.5   ADH is composed of a uniform population of cells that are evenly distributed within the micropapillae, which extend to the basement membrane rather than being "perched" on the surface of the luminal epithelial layer.

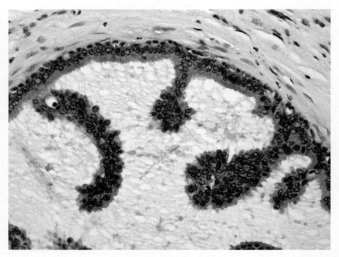

Figure 4.2.10   The micropapillae of DCIS are bulbous and are attached to the basement membrane.

	Micropapillary DCIS	Usual Hyperplasia Resembling Gynecomastia
Age	Adult women	Adult women
Location	Anywhere in the breast	Anywhere in the breast
Imaging findings	Calcifications, rarely mass or nipple discharge	Calcifications, often incidental finding
Etiology	Unknown	Unknown
Histology	1. Micropapillary proliferation involving several expanded lobular units and ducts *(Figs. 4.3.1–4.3.6)* 2. Proliferation of uniform cells evenly placed within bulbous micropapillae *(Figs. 4.3.5 and 4.3.6)* 3. Micropapillae lack fibrovascular cores and extend into the lumen from the basement membrane *(Figs. 4.3.5 and 4.3.6)* 4. May be of low, intermediate, or high nuclear grade 5. May be present in a patchy distribution within individual lobular units; however, involvement of numerous spaces supports a diagnosis of micropapillary DCIS *(Figs. 4.3.1 and 4.3.2)*	1. Epithelial proliferation within terminal duct lobular units *(Figs. 4.3.7–4.3.12)* 2. Cellular variability and indistinct cell borders characteristic 3. Small bland cells with pyknotic nuclei form tapering, "pinched-appearing" micropapillary projections *(Figs. 4.3.10–4.3.12)* 4. Micropapillary projections appear "stuck on" luminal layer *(Fig. 4.3.12)*
Special studies	None; CK5/6 usually not expressed; ER expression routinely assessed to predict response to adjuvant endocrine therapy following a diagnosis of DCIS; multigene assay may predict which patients may be spared radiation	None; CK 5/6 may show patchy expression
Genetic abnormalities	Loss of 16q, 17p	None
Treatment	Complete excision with negative margins, ± adjuvant radiation, ± antiestrogen therapy; sentinel lymph node biopsy not indicated; pure micropapillary DCIS may be extensively present in the breast, requiring mastectomy	Excision not necessary when detected in core biopsy specimen
Clinical implication	Development of invasive carcinoma in approximately 30% of cases if incompletely excised; with complete excision, recurrence rate approximately 5%–8% without radiation; recurrence rate less than 5% for low grade DCIS of limited extent	Slightly increased risk of later cancer development (1.5×); risk is bilateral, but of insufficient magnitude to affect patient management

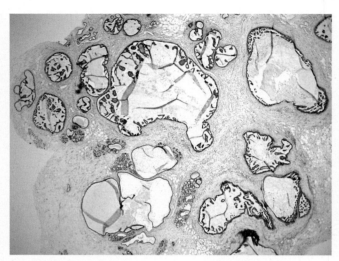

Figure 4.3.1   Several adjacent lobular units are expanded by an epithelial proliferation that forms micropapillae, imparting a "shaggy" appearance to the spaces in DCIS.

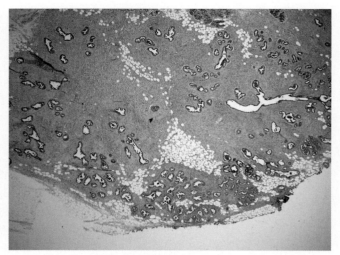

Figure 4.3.7   Hyperplasia resembling gynecomastia forms a nodule of fibrous stroma containing an epithelial proliferation.

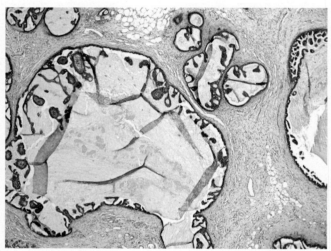

Figure 4.3.2   Bulbous micropapillae of DCIS project from the basement membrane and some appear unattached within the lumen.

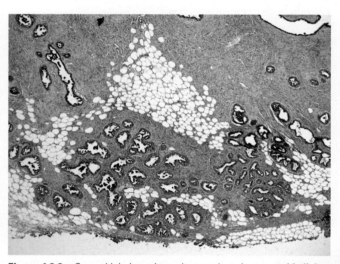

Figure 4.3.8   Several lobular units and a true duct show an epithelial proliferation forming micropapillary structures in hyperplasia resembling gynecomastia.

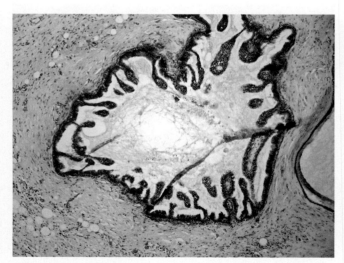

Figure 4.3.3   Some of the micropapillae are fused in this example of DCIS.

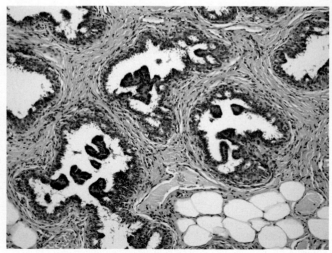

Figure 4.3 9   Stromal changes accompany the epithelial hyperplasia; intralobular stroma is fibrous, similar to pseudoangiomatous stromal hyperplasia.

4 Ductal Carcinoma In Situ

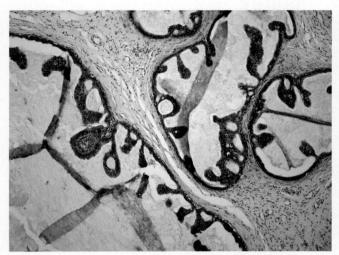

Figure 4.3.4   Micropapillary DCIS characteristically has a patchy distribution, with some spaces partially involved by micropapillae; however, the non-micropapillary luminal epithelium has the same cytology as the micropapillae.

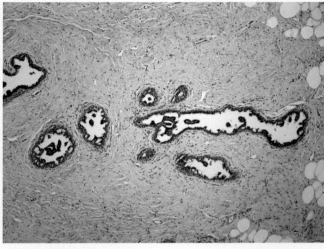

Figure 4.3.10   Micropapillae are focally present in true ducts as well as in lobular units in hyperplasia resembling gynecomastia.

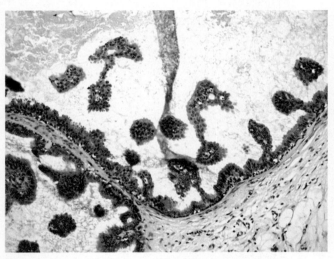

Figure 4.3.5   Detached micropapillae within the lumen highlight the 3-dimensional complexity of micropapillary DCIS.

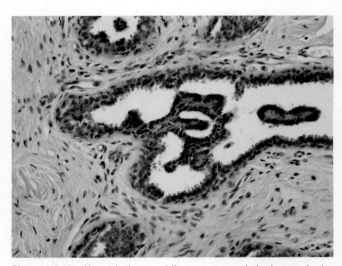

Figure 4.3.11   Hyperplasia resembling gynectomastia is characterized by cells with pyknotic nuclei peripherally arranged around micropapillae with "empty" centers.

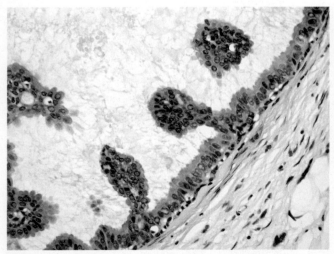

Figure 4.3.6   Micropapillae of DCIS may appear tapered near the point of attachment; however, neoplastic cells are evenly distributed around the bulbous projections. Note similarity of the lining epithelium to that forming the micropapillae.

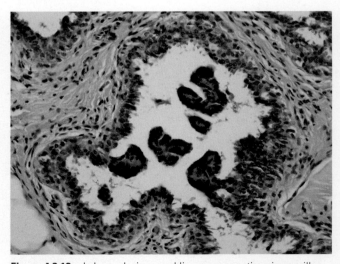

Figure 4.3.12   In hyperplasia resembling gynecomastia, micropapillae composed of cells with pyknotic nuclei appear "stuck" on the luminal epithelium, without connection to the basement membrane. The lining epithelium shows nuclear variability.

	Intermediate-Grade DCIS	Florid Hyperplasia without Atypia
Age	Adult women, usually 50 y or older	Adult women
Location	Anywhere in the breast	Anywhere in the breast
Imaging findings	Calcifications, rarely mass-forming	Calcifications, rarely mass-forming often incidental
Etiology	Unknown	Unknown
Histology	1. Terminal ducts as well as true ducts are involved by epithelial proliferation *(Figs. 4.4.1–4.4.4)* 2. Initial impression of nuclear overlap; however, nuclei resemble each other, without true variability *(Figs. 4.4.3 and 4.4.4)* 3. Intermediate-grade nuclei that appear "frozen in place" without streaming or swirling *(Figs. 4.4.3 and 4.4.4)* 4. Subtle microrosettes are frequently present *(Fig. 4.4.4)*	1. Affects terminal duct lobular unit *(Figs. 4.4.5–4.4.8)* 2. Nuclear variability and overlap *(Figs. 4.4.7 and 4.4.8)* 3. Irregular secondary spaces *(Fig. 4.4.6)* 4. Indistinct cell borders *(Fig. 4.4.8)*
Special studies	None; CK5/6 usually not expressed; ER expression routinely assessed to predict response to adjuvant endocrine therapy; multigene assay may predict which patients may be spared radiation	None; CK5/6 is variably expressed
Genetic abnormalities	Loss of 16q, 17p	None
Treatment	Complete excision with negative margins, ± adjuvant radiation, ± antiestrogen therapy	None
Clinical implication	Development of invasive carcinoma in approximately 30% of cases if incompletely excised; with complete excision, recurrence rate approximately 5%–8% for DCIS of limited extent	Slightly increased risk of later cancer development (1.5×) in either breast; risk level insufficient to affect patient management

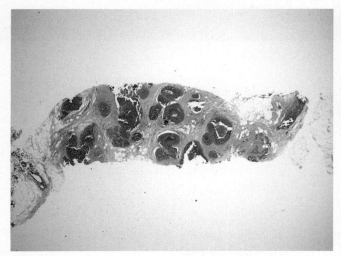

Figure 4.4.1   DCIS: Core needle biopsy specimen showing several lobular units and intervening ducts containing a solid epithelial proliferation with necrosis.

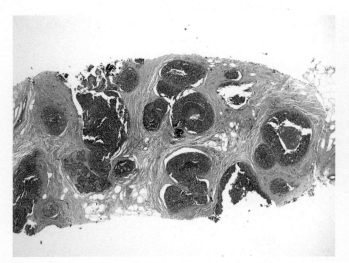

Figure 4.4.2   A papilloma is present (left of center), showing the same proliferation as the surrounding ducts in this example of DCIS.

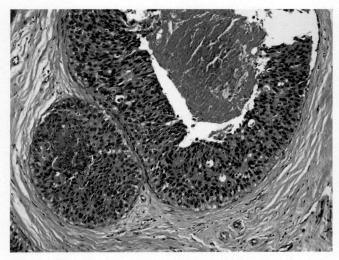

Figure 4.4.3   Although there is a suggestion of nuclear streaming and swirling, cellular monotony is characteristic of DCIS.

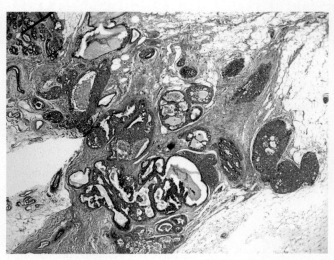

Figure 4.4.5   A solid epithelial proliferation involves adjacent lobular units in florid hyperplasia without atypia.

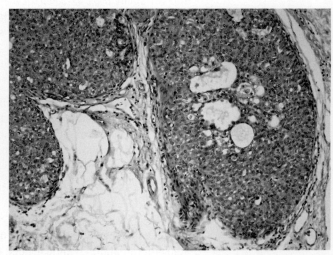

Figure 4.4.6   Nuclear variability, cellular overlap, and irregular secondary spaces characterize florid hyperplasia without atypia.

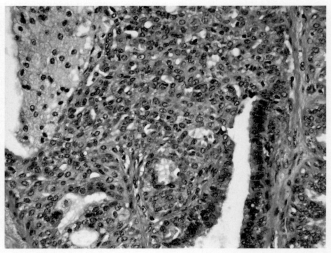

Figure 4.4.7   Florid hyperplasia without atypia has irregular secondary spaces and indistinct cell borders.

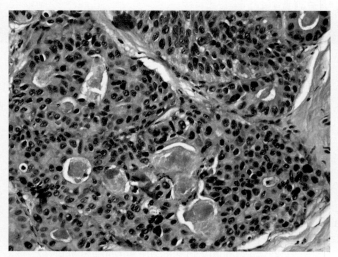

Figure 4.4.4 Subtle microrosettes formed by uniform cells characterize this pattern of DCIS. The cells of adjacent microrosettes appear to overlap, but they are evenly distributed around their respective secondary spaces.

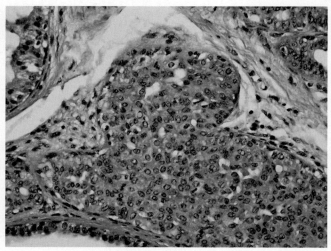

Figure 4.4.8 Nuclear variability and occasional inclusions "heliotropes" are a defining feature of florid hyperplasia without atypia.

	Spindle Cell Pattern DCIS	Usual Hyperplasia without Atypia
Age	Adult women, usually 50 y or older	Adult women
Location	Anywhere in the breast	Anywhere in the breast
Imaging findings	Calcifications, rarely mass-forming	Calcifications or incidental
Etiology	Unknown	Unknown
Histology	1. Terminal ducts as well as true ducts are expanded by a solid epithelial proliferation *(Figs. 4.5.1–4.5.3)* 2. Initial impression of nuclear overlap; however, cells resemble each other, without true variability *(Fig. 4.5.4)* 3. Epithelial proliferation is composed of low to intermediate grade nuclei that show spindled morphology with occasional microrosettes *(Figs. 4.5.5 and 4.5.6)*	1. Nuclear variability, swirling or streaming pattern, nuclear overlap 2. Secondary spaces are peripheral and irregular. 3. Epithelial proliferation may be solid without secondary spaces *(Figs. 4.5.7–4.5.11)*
Special studies	None; CK5/6 usually not expressed; ER expression routinely assessed to predict response to adjuvant endocrine therapy; multigene assay may predict which patients may be spared radiation	None, CK5/6 is variably expressed
Genetic abnormalities	None specific to the spindle cell pattern	None
Treatment	Complete excision with negative margins, ± adjuvant radiation, ± antiestrogen therapy; sentinel lymph node biopsy not indicated	Excision not necessary if detected on core biopsy specimen
Clinical implication	Development of invasive carcinoma in approximately 30% of cases if incompletely excised; with complete excision, recurrence rate approximately 5%–8% without radiation	Slightly increased risk of later cancer development (1.5×); insufficient to affect patient management

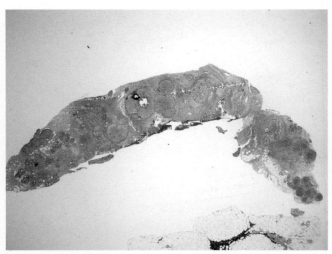

Figure 4.5.1   DCIS: Core biopsy showing distended and distorted lobular units, terminal and true ducts with calcification.

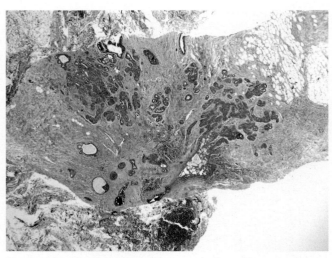

Figure 4.5.7   Usual hyperplasia without atypia: A core biopsy showing two adjacent lobular units and a terminal duct with an epithelial proliferation.

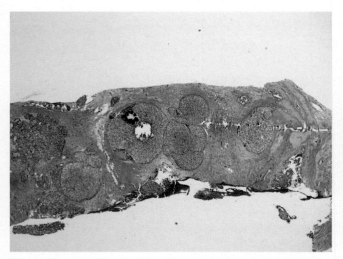

Figure 4.5.2   A solid epithelial proliferation involves essentially all of the epithelium in this core biopsy specimen containing DCIS.

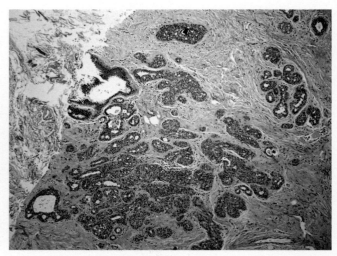

Figure 4.5.8   Epithelial distention and distortion are mild; focal apocrine change is present in this example of usual hyperplasia without atypia. Note intercellular spaces with irregular contours are evident at low power, an important clue to a benign proliferative process.

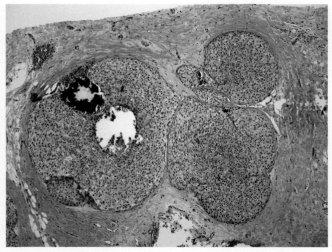

Figure 4.5.3   True ducts are markedly distended by spindled DCIS cells with uniform nuclei and associated calcification.

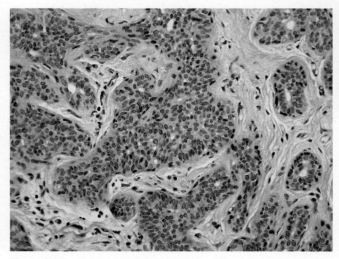

Figure 4.5.9   Nuclear variability, indistinct cell borders, and uneven cell placement are characteristic of usual hyperplasia without atypia.

4 Ductal Carcinoma In Situ

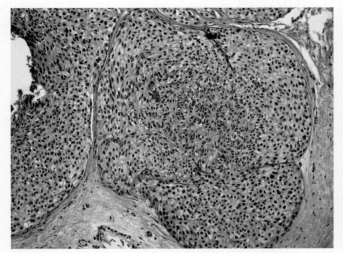

Figure 4.5.4   The spindled DCIS cells appear to be arranged in a streaming or swirling pattern centrally, mimicking florid hyperplasia.

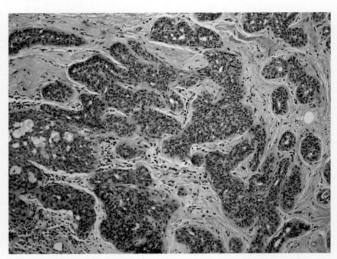

Figure 4.5.10   Usual hyperplasia without atypia has irregular secondary spaces.

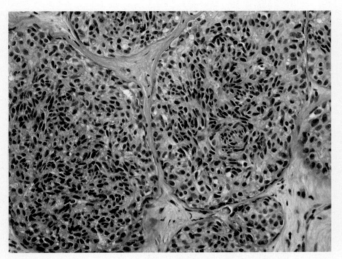

Figure 4.5.5   Both nuclei and cytoplasm are uniform in DCIS, and the apparent second population of cells is the spindled cells cut in cross section.

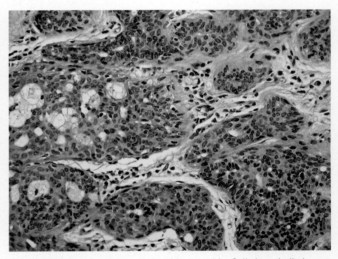

Figure 4.5.11   Usual hyperplasia without atypia: Cells have indistinct cell borders, nuclei are variable, and secondary spaces are irregular.

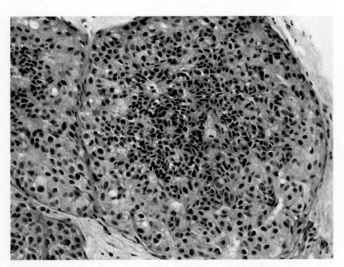

Figure 4.5.6   Subtle microrosettes are formed by the spindle cells in this pattern of DCIS.

	Apocrine Ductal Carcinoma In Situ	Apocrine Atypical Ductal Hyperplasia
Age	Adult women	Adult women
Location	Anywhere in the breast	Anywhere in the breast
Imaging findings	Calcifications, rarely a mass	Calcifications or incidental
Etiology	Unknown	Unknown
Histology	1. Apocrine cells with rigid architecture, or solid growth *(Figs. 4.6.1–4.6.5)* 2. Pattern composed of evenly placed cells *(Fig. 4.6.5)*; may show patchy involvement of ducts and lobular units 3. May be of low, intermediate, or high nuclear grade	1. Uniform apocrine cells with low-grade nuclei *(Figs. 4.6.6–4.6.10)* 2. Rigid secondary spaces or solid proliferation with even cell placement *(Figs. 4.6.8, 4.6.10)* 3. Limited to partial involvement of terminal duct/lobular unit *(Fig. 4.6.10)*
Special studies	Expresses androgen receptor (AR); usually ER-negative	None
Genetic abnormalities	Overexpression of AR mRNA and of genes downstream in the AR pathway; *FOXA1* mRNA overexpression; absence of *ESR1* mRNA overexpression	Unknown
Treatment	Excision with negative margins, ± radiation therapy, ± antiestrogen therapy	Excision if detected in core biopsy specimen; mammographic follow-up ± antiestrogen therapy
Clinical implication	Apocrine DCIS may be extensive with patchy involvement of lobular units, which has implications for margin assessment	Moderately increased risk of later cancer development (4–5×); risk is bilateral

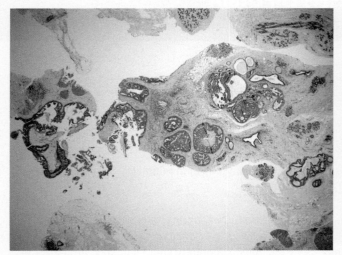

Figure 4.6.1 Apocrine DCIS: A core biopsy specimen contains an epithelial proliferation that involves several contiguous ducts and lobular units.

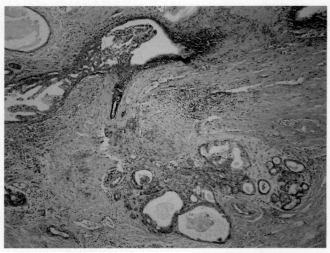

Figure 4.6.6 ADH with apocrine cytology: A terminal duct and an adjacent lobular unit are partially involved by an apocrine proliferation.

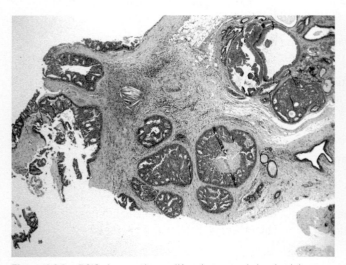

Figure 4.6.2 DCIS: An apocrine proliferation expands involved ducts and lobular units.

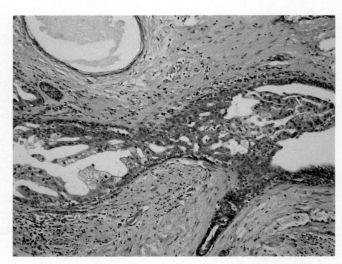

Figure 4.6.7 Apocrine ADH has foci of uniform cells including rare micropapillary projections; note second normal population of cells at the periphery of the duct (right).

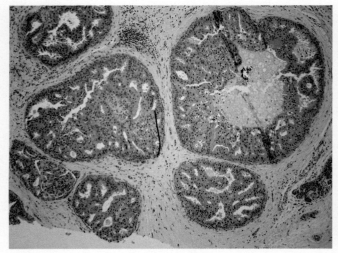

Figure 4.6.3 Secondary spaces are slightly irregular but have rigid architecture with cribriform structures in apocrine DCIS.

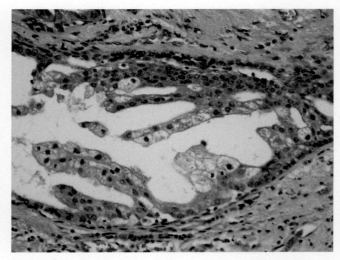

Figure 4.6.8 A terminal duct contains an apocrine proliferation showing even cell placement, micropapillary projections, and uniform nuclei qualifying as ADH; normal peripheral cells are present.

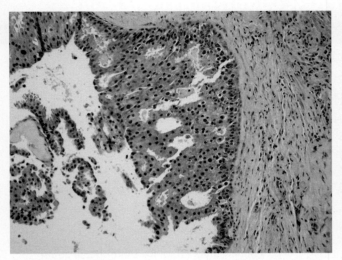

Figure 4.6.4 A uniform population of apocrine cells is evenly placed in DCIS and forms round secondary spaces.

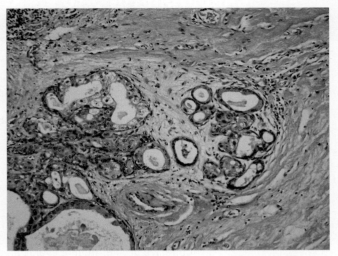

Figure 4.6.9 A lobular unit is partially involved by atypical apocrine cells in this example of ADH.

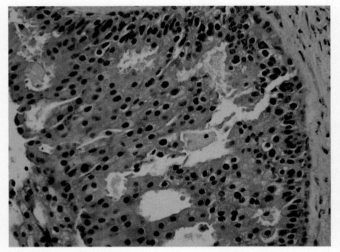

Figure 4.6.5 Low-grade DCIS (apocrine type): Cells are uniform throughout the proliferation, which qualifies as DCIS given the extent of the contiguously involved spaces.

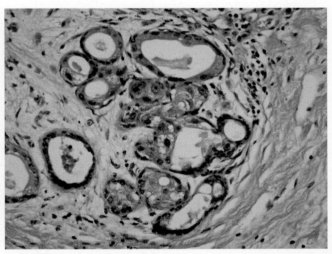

Figure 4.6.10 ADH involving a lobular unit. Most acini of this lobular unit contain atypical apocrine cells and residual normal epithelium.

4 Ductal Carcinoma In Situ

	Lobular Unit Involvement by Low-Grade DCIS	Atypical Lobular Hyperplasia (ALH)
Age	Adult women, incidence increases with age	Adult women, incidence drops following menopause
Location	Anywhere in the breast	Anywhere in the breast
Imaging findings	Calcifications, rarely mass-forming	Incidental finding, rarely associated with calcification
Etiology	Unknown	Unknown
Histology	1. Cohesive proliferation of evenly placed uniform cells involving ducts and lobular units *(Figs. 4.7.1–4.7.5)* 2. Distinct cell borders *(Figs. 4.7.4–4.7.5)*	1. Lobular units contain a uniform cell population, with some filling of acini by small cells with a dyshesive growth pattern *(Figs. 4.7.6–4.7.9)* 2. Acini contain characteristic cells, but are not fully distended or distorted *(Figs. 4.7.6–4.7.9)* 3. Residual luminal epithelial and myoepithelial cells are present *(Figs. 4.7.6–4.7.9)* 4. Intracytoplasmic lumens are common *(Fig. 4.7.9)*
Special studies	None required; strong uniform E-cadherin expression; CK5/6 usually not expressed; ER expression routinely assessed to predict response to adjuvant endocrine therapy following a diagnosis of DCIS; multigene assay may predict which patients may be spared radiation	None; E-cadherin is usually not expressed; p120 expression maintained
Genetic abnormalities	Loss of 16q, 17p	Mutations of *CDH1* (chromosome 16q22.1)
Treatment	Excision to negative margins, ± radiation, ± antiestrogen therapy	Excision not required if incidental finding on core biopsy; mammographic follow-up ± antiestrogen therapy
Clinical implication	Eventuate in invasive carcinoma in approximately 30% of cases if incompletely excised; with complete excision, recurrence rate approximately 5%–8% without radiation; Recurrence rate <5% for low grade DCIS of limited extent	Moderately increased risk of later cancer development (4–5×); bilateral risk, with ipsilateral breast at greater (3:1) risk

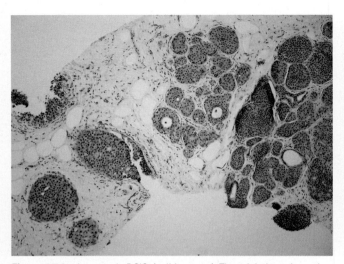

Figure 4.7.1   Low-grade DCIS, (solid pattern): Three lobular units and a terminal duct contain a uniform cellular proliferation.

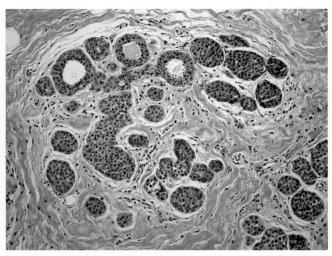

Figure 4.7.6   ALH: Two lobular units contain a proliferation of uniform cells with a few lumens remaining.

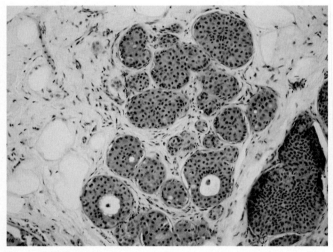

Figure 4.7.2   Acini and a terminal duct contain round, regular cells that are evenly placed in this example of DCIS.

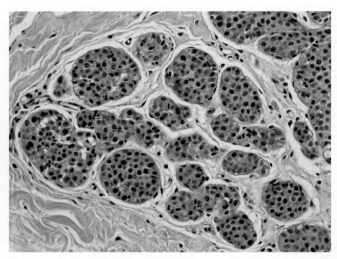

Figure 4.7.7   Cells of ALH are round and regular with cellular dyshesion.

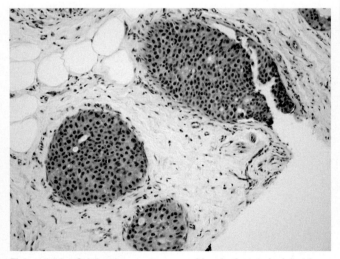

Figure 4.7.3   Subtle microrosettes are evident in the terminal duct in this example of low grade DCIS.

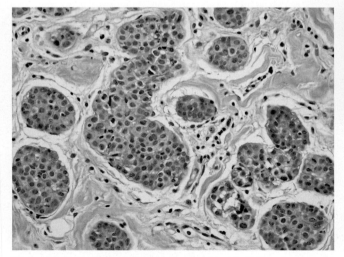

Figure 4.7.8   Lack of cellular cohesion is evident in ALH.

4 Ductal Carcinoma In Situ

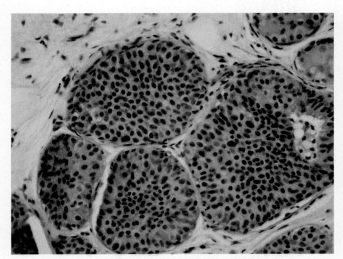

Figure 4.7.4   Neoplastic cells are cohesive and lack intracytoplasmic inclusions in low grade, solid pattern DCIS.

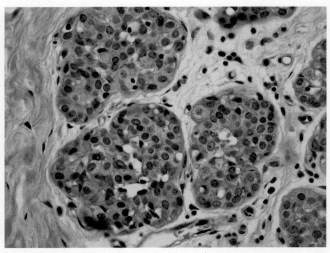

Figure 4.7.9   Cellular characteristics of lobular neoplasia include bland nuclei, dyshesive growth pattern, and occasional intracytoplasmic inclusions.

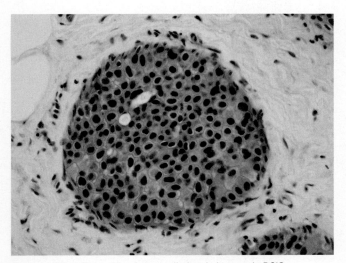

Figure 4.7.5   The cell borders are distinct in low grade DCIS.

	Pagetoid DCIS	Ductal involvement by Lobular Neoplasia
Age	Adult women, incidence increases with age	Adult women, incidence drops following menopause
Location	Anywhere in the breast	Anywhere in the breast
Imaging findings	Calcifications, rarely mass-forming, may be associated with nipple discharge	Incidental finding, rarely associated with calcifications
Etiology	Unknown	Unknown
Histology	1. Terminal and large duct involvement with patchy involvement of adjacent lobular units *(Fig. 4.8.1)* 2. Cohesive neoplastic epithelium undermines normal luminal epithelium *(Figs. 4.8.2–4.8.4)*	1. Lobular neoplasia cells spread along terminal ducts; occasionally true ducts are involved *(Figs. 4.8.5–4.8.8)* 2. Cells are small, round, and regular; intracytoplasmic inclusions frequent *(Fig. 4.8.8)* 3. Adjacent acini show similar cells with a dyshesive growth pattern, either as ALH or lobular carcinoma in situ (LCIS) *(Figs. 4.8.5–4.8.7)* 4. Residual luminal epithelial cells overlie or are interspersed among lobular neoplasia cells *(Figs. 4.8.7 and 4.8.8)*
Special studies	Neoplastic cells express E-cadherin, and often overexpress HER2 (a reflection of cellular motility); ER expression routinely assessed to predict response to adjuvant endocrine therapy	None; E-cadherin shows reduced or absent expression; p120 expression maintained
Genetic abnormalities	Loss of 16q, 17p	Mutations of *CDH1* (chromosome 16q22.1)
Treatment	Excision to negative margins, ± radiation, ± antiestrogen therapy	Excision not required if incidental finding on core biopsy; mammographic follow-up ± antiestrogen therapy
Clinical implication	Pagetoid DCIS may be extensive with patchy involvement of lobular units, which has implications for margin assessment	Moderately increased risk of later cancer development (4–5×); bilateral risk with ipsilateral breast at greater (3:1) risk

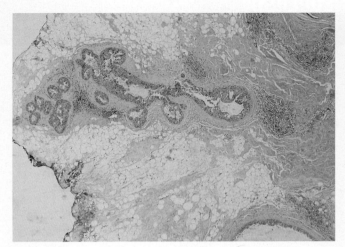

Figure 4.8.1   A terminal duct and adjacent lobular unit contain an epithelial proliferation. Pagetoid DCIS often partially involves lobular units without distortion.

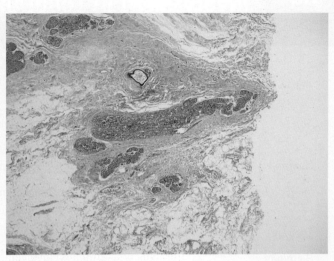

Figure 4.8.5   A terminal duct and several adjacent lobular units contain an epithelial proliferation. The single true duct is not involved in this example of ALH.

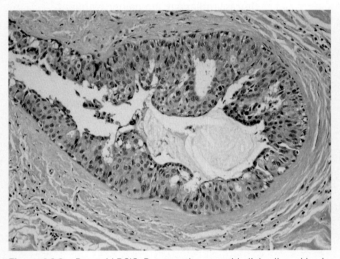

Figure 4.8.2   Pagetoid DCIS: Between the myoepithelial cells and luminal epithelium there is a proliferation of evenly placed, uniform cells with distinct cell borders.

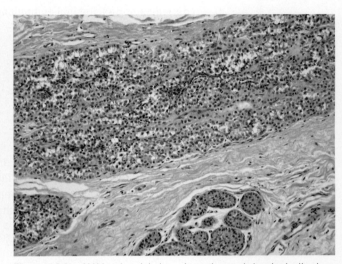

Figure 4.8.6   ALH involves lobular units and spreads longitudually along the terminal duct.

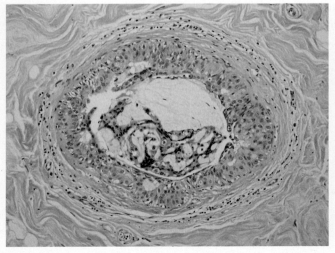

Figure 4.8.3   Residual luminal epithelium should not be interpreted as cellular variability, i.e., usual hyperplasia, in this example of Pagetoid DCIS.

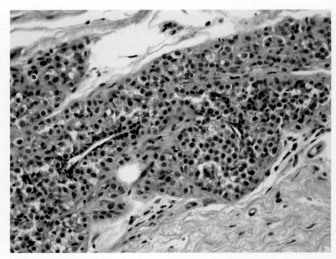

Figure 4.8.7   A small amount of residual luminal epithelium is present. A dyshesive growth pattern is evident in ALH.

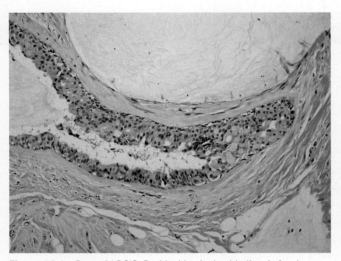

Figure 4.8.4   Pagetoid DCIS: Residual luminal epithelium is focal.

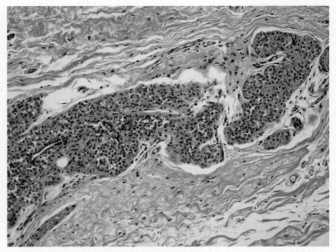

Figure 4.8.8   Small round cells with intracytoplasmic inclusions, have the dyshesive growth pattern defining of ALH. Focally normal luminal epithelium remains.

	Low-Grade DCIS	Classic LCIS
Age	Adult women, usually 55 y and older	Adult women, incidence drops following menopause
Location	Anywhere in the breast	Anywhere in the breast
Imaging findings	Usually calcifications, rarely mass-forming	Incidental finding, rarely associated with calcification
Etiology	Unknown	Unknown
Histology	1. Complete involvement of at least 2 adjacent spaces, usually with true duct involvement, extending over an area of at least 3.0 mm *(Fig. 4.9.1)* 2. Uniform cell population, distinct cell borders, even cell placement, solid growth pattern with subtle microrosettes *(Figs. 4.9.2–4.9.6)*	1. Uniform cell population with distention and distortion of involved spaces *(Figs. 4.9.6–4.9.9)* 2. Dyshesive growth pattern *(Fig. 4.9.9)* 3. Intracytoplasmic lumens are characteristic *(Fig. 4.9.9)* 4. Often shows Pagetoid spread in terminal ducts *(Fig. 4.9.10)*
Special studies	None; strong uniform E-cadherin expression *(Fig. 4.9.4)*; CK5/6 usually not expressed; ER expression routinely assessed to predict response to adjuvant endocrine therapy; multigene assay may predict which patients may be spared radiation	Loss of E-cadherin expression *(Fig. 4.9.9)*; p120 expression maintained
Genetic abnormalities	Loss of 16q, 17p	Mutations of *CDH1* (chromosome 16q22.1)
Treatment	Excision to negative margins, ± radiation, ± antiestrogen therapy	Mammographic follow-up ± antiestrogen therapy; usually excised if detected on core biopsy specimen
Clinical implication	Eventuates in invasive carcinoma in approximately 30% of cases if not completely excised; with complete excision, recurrence rate approximately 5%–8% without radiation; for low-grade DCIS of limited extent recurrence rates <5%	High risk (9–10×) of later cancer development; bilateral risk with ipsilateral breast at greatest risk (3:1); risk drops following menopause

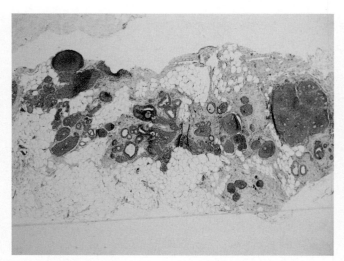

Figure 4.9.1 This example of low-grade DCIS contains a solid and cribriform epithelial proliferation that involves several lobular units and terminal ducts.

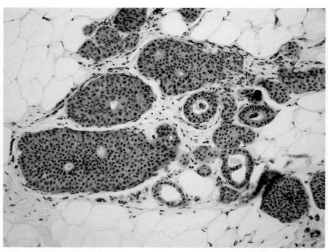

Figure 4.9.2 Acini are expanded by a uniform population of cells with distinct cell borders.

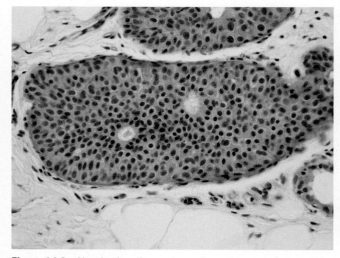

Figure 4.9.3 Neoplastic cells are arranged as numerous microrosettes, characteristic of low-grade DCIS.

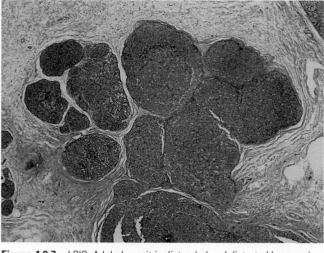

Figure 4.9.7 LCIS: A lobular unit is distended and distorted by an epithelial proliferation which also involves the terminal duct.

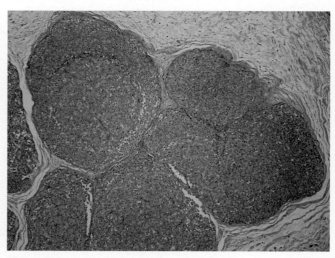

Figure 4.9.8 Acini are markedly distended in LCIS.

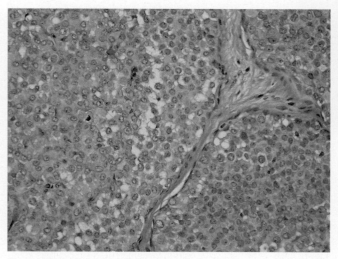

Figure 4.9.9 Cells of LCIS are small, round and often contain intracytoplasmic inclusions. A dyshesive growth pattern is evident.

4 Ductal Carcinoma In Situ

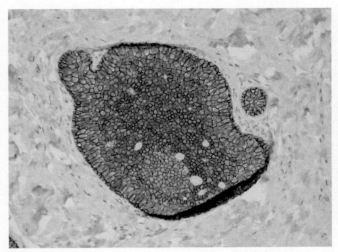

Figure 4.9.4   An E-cadherin immunohistochemical study shows strong membranous expression in low-grade DCIS.

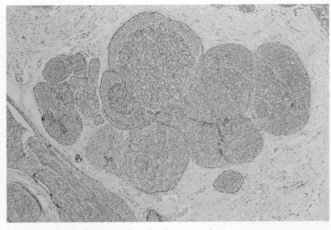

Figure 4.9.10   LCIS lacks E-cadherin expression.

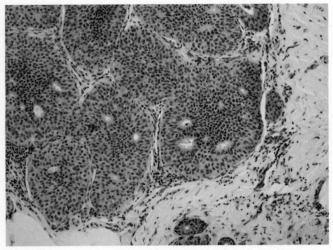

Figure 4.9.5   A monotonous cell population expands the involved spaces of low-grade DCIS; a second population of cells is lacking.

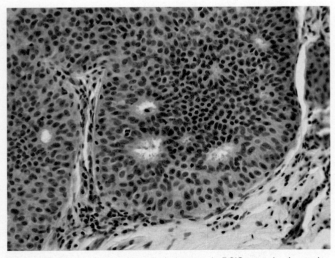

Figure 4.9.6   The neoplastic cells in low grade DCIS are cohesive and appear "frozen in space".

	DCIS with Lobular Cytology	Classic LCIS
Age	Adult women, incidence increases with age	Adult women, incidence drops following menopause
Location	Anywhere in the breast	Anywhere in the breast
Imaging findings	Calcifications, often mass-forming	Incidental finding, rarely associated with calcification
Etiology	Unknown	Unknown
Histology	1. Dense disease usually involving several lobular units and true ducts *(Fig. 4.10.1–4.10.5)* 2. Solid growth pattern with central necrosis and calcification *(Figs. 4.10.2 and 4.10.3)* 3. Usually intermediate or high nuclear grade *(Fig. 4.10.4)* 4. May show Pagetoid spread and focally dyshesive growth pattern *(Fig. 4.10.5)*	1. Small, round uniform cell population with dyshesive growth pattern *(Fig. 4.10.6–4.10.8)* 2. Intracytoplasmic lumens *(Fig. 4.10.8)* 3. Marked distention and distortion of involved acini *(Fig. 4.10.7)* 4. Often with Pagetoid spread *(Fig. 4.10.6)*
Special studies	None required; variable CK5/6 expression; variable ER expression; high grade DCIS often lacks ER expression; may lack or have reduced E-cadherin expression	Loss of E-cadherin expression; p120 expression maintained
Genetic abnormalities	Unknown	Mutations of *CDH1* (chromosome 16q22.1)
Treatment	Excision with adequate margins, ± radiation, ± antiestrogen therapy	Mammographic follow-up ± antiestrogen therapy; usually excised if detected on core biopsy specimen
Clinical implication	Eventuates in invasive carcinoma in approximately 30% of cases if not completely excised. Density of disease and growth pattern involving true ducts supports clinical behavior as DCIS, requiring DCIS treatment.	High risk (9–10×) of later cancer development; bilateral risk with ipsilateral breast at greatest risk (3:1); risk drops following menopause

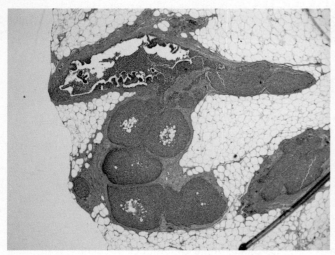

Figure 4.10.1   DCIS: Two lobular units and a true duct show marked distention.

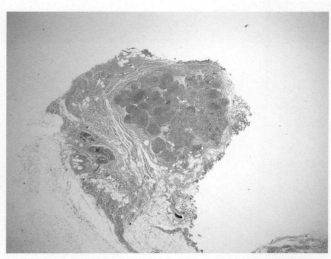

Figure 4.10.6   The majority of the acini of this lobular unit show distention and distortion diagnostic of LCIS.

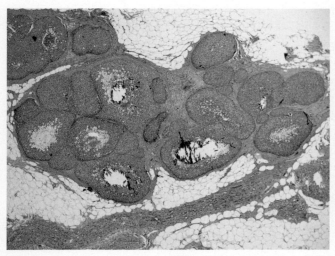

Figure 4.10.2   This unit contains a solid proliferation associated with central necrosis and calcification in this example of DCIS.

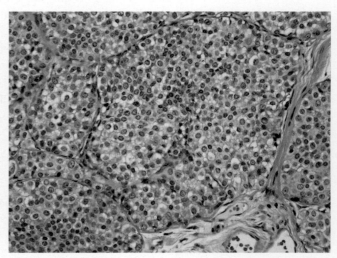

Figure 4.10.7   The cells of LCIS are small, round and regular.

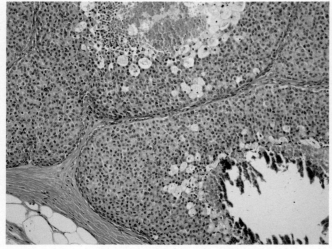

Figure 4.10.3   Acini are markedly distorted by the DCIS cells.

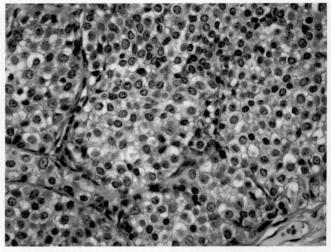

Figure 4.10.8   A dyshesive growth pattern, bland nuclei and occasional intracytoplasmic inclusions are characteristic of classic LCIS.

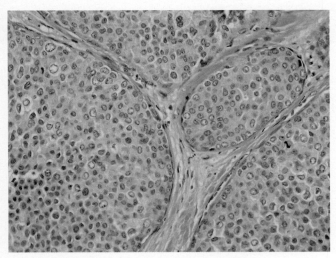

Figure 4.10.4   A solid growth pattern composed of cells having intermediate-grade nuclei is diagnostic for DCIS.

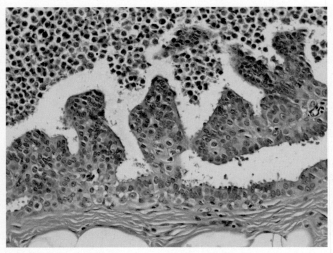

Figure 4.10.5   Neoplastic cells show Pagetoid spread along this true duct in this example of DCIS with lobular cytology.

	Secretory Pattern DCIS	Secretory Change
Age	Adult women	Adult women, any age
Location	Anywhere in the breast	Anywhere in the breast
Imaging findings	Calcification, rarely mass-forming	Calcification
Etiology	Unknown	Idiopathic, or may be associated with prolactin-producing pituitary adenoma or some drugs
Histology	1. Lobular units, terminal and true ducts involved by an epithelial proliferation with clear cytoplasm *(Figs. 4.11.1–4.11.4)* 2. Secretory material rather than necrosis is present centrally in the involved space *(Fig. 4.11.2)* 3. Cellular uniformity is evident despite the suggestion of uneven cell placement *(Figs. 4.11.3 and 4.11.4)* 4. Cells form glandular structures	1. Affects lobular units and terminal ducts *(Figs.4.11.5–4.11.8)* 2. Mild epithelial proliferation (one or two cell layers) of hobnail cells with enlarged nuclei and bubbly cytoplasm *(Figs. 4.11.5–4.11.8)* 3. Lumens often contain secretory material with spherical calcifications *(Fig. 4.11.6)* 4. Cytologic changes similar to Arias Stella reaction *(Fig. 4.11.6–4.11.8)*
Special studies	None required; variable CK5/6 expression; variable ER expression; ER expression routinely assessed to predict response to adjuvant endocrine therapy; multigene assay may predict which patients may be spared radiation	None
Genetic abnormalities	Unknown	None
Treatment	Excision with negative margins, ± radiation, ± antiestrogen therapy	Excision is not indicated if detected in a core biopsy specimen
Clinical Implication	Eventuate in invasive carcinoma in approximately 30% of cases if incompletely excised	No association with cancer risk or more concerning lesions

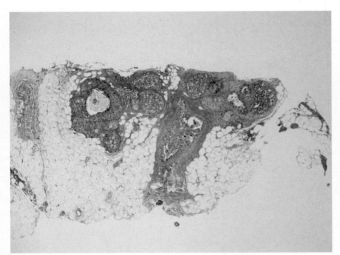

Figure 4.11.1   A core biopsy specimen shows an epithelial proliferation affecting two lobular units and a terminal duct in this example of secretory type DCIS.

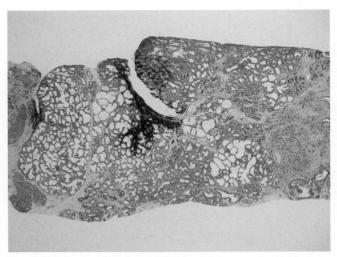

Figure 4.11.5   Several adjacent lobular units are expanded in this example of secretory change.

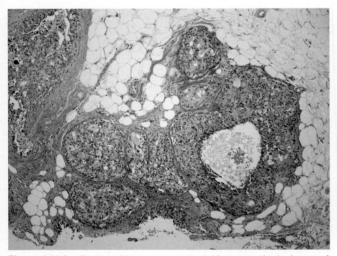

Figure 4.11.2   Eosinophilic secretory material is present in the lumen of an involved acinus.

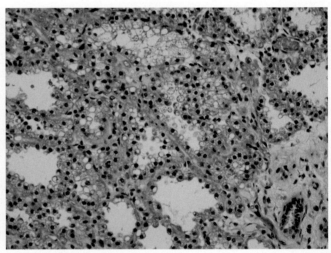

Figure 4.11.6   In addition to lobular units, a terminal duct is also involved by secretory change.

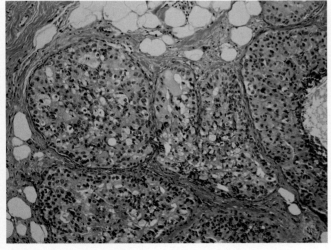

Figure 4.11.3   The neoplastic cells of DCIS are arranged around glandular structures, suggesting uneven cell placement.

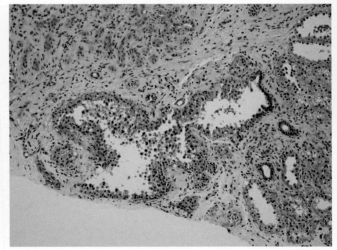

Figure 4.11.7   Secretory change: Cells have bubbly cytoplasm, a hobnail configuration, and slightly enlarged nuclei.

4 Ductal Carcinoma In Situ

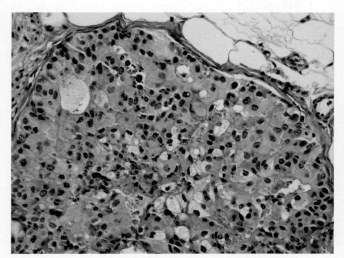

Figure 4.11.4   Cells have intermediate-grade nuclei, are arranged in rosettes and have cytoplasmic vacuoles and secretory material.

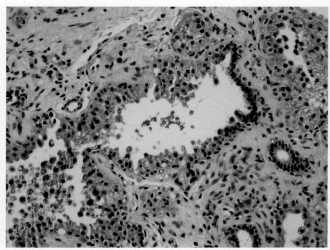

Figure 4.11.8   Secretory material is present in lumens. Mild nuclear enlargement should not be interpreted as atypia.

	Paget Disease	Prominent Toker Cells
Age	Adult women	Adult women
Location	Skin of the nipple	Skin of the nipple
Imaging findings	No findings specific to Paget disease, although when associated with underlying carcinoma, a mass and/or calcifications may be present	None
Etiology	Unknown	Unknown
Histology	1. Malignant cells spread singly or in small groups along the dermal epidermal junction with upward migration in epidermis *(Figs. 4.12.1 and 4.12.2)* 2. Cells with ample cytoplasm contain enlarged nuclei, many of which have prominent nucleoli *(Fig. 4.12.2)* 3. Malignant cells are separated from the surrounding squamous epithelium by pale halos *(Fig. 4.12.2)*	1. Pale, bland single cells within epidermis *(Figs. 4.12.4 and 4.12.5)*, normal constituent of skin of nipple 2. Round to ovoid nuclei with smooth contours and amorphous chromatin *(Fig. 4.12.5)*
Special studies	Positive for expression of CK7; HER2 overexpression in more than 90% of cases (a reflection of cellular motility) *(Fig. 4.12.3)*	Negative for expression of CK7; HER2 negative
Genetic Abnormalities	No recurrent alteration specific to Paget disease; genetic alterations mirror underlying carcinoma when present	None
Treatment	Complete excision of Paget component; treat any underling carcinoma component as appropriate	None
Clinical implication	Underlying DCIS or invasive carcinoma present in more than 95% of cases; ulceration associated with Paget disease does not qualify as pT4b	None

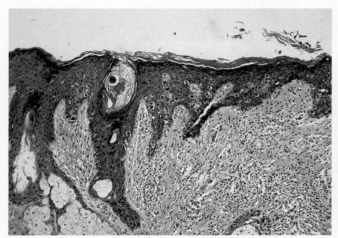

Figure 4.12.1   Paget disease of the nipple characterized by malignant cells spreading singly or in small groups along the dermal–epidermal junction with upward migration within the epidermis.

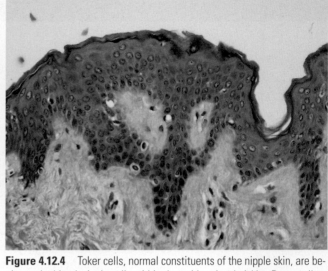

Figure 4.12.4   Toker cells, normal constituents of the nipple skin, are benign, pale, bland, single cells within the epidermis mimicking Paget cells.

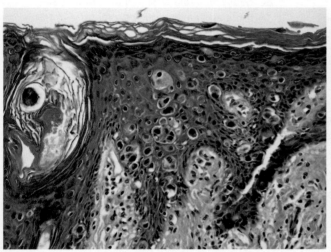

Figure 4.12.2   Nuclei of the Paget cells are large and atypical with prominent nucleoli. These malignant cells are separated from the surrounding squamous epithelium by pale halos.

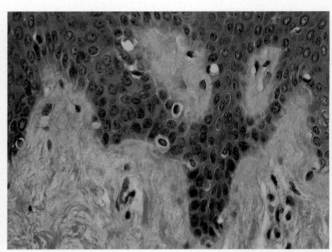

Figure 4.12.5   Toker cells have round to ovoid nuclei with smooth contours and amorphous chromatin.

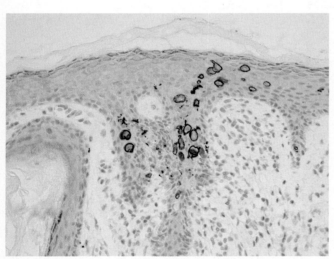

Figure 4.12.3   Paget cells showing over-expression of HER2 (strong circumferential membranous staining).

	DCIS in a Background of Hypersecretory Hyperplasia	Hypersecretory Hyperplasia
Age	Adult women, usually 55 y or older	Adult women
Location	Anywhere in the breast	Anywhere in the breast
Imaging findings	Calcifications, rarely mass-forming	Calcifications in clusters, may be pleomorphic
Etiology	Unknown	Unknown
Histology	1. Extensive and monotonous epithelial proliferation with numerous intraluminal projections which involves many lobular units and true ducts *(Fig. 4.13.1)* 2. The malignant nuclei are multilayered and monotonous, forming numerous complex intraluminal papillary projections *(Fig. 4.13.2)* 3. Uniform cells with intermediate-grade nuclei and prominent nucleoli are diagnostic of DCIS *(Fig. 4.13.3)* 4. Solid pattern growth may be focal *(Fig. 4.13.4)*	1. Enlarged lobular units composed of variably dilated acini containing abundant secretory material associated with calcifications *(Figs. 4.13.5–4.13.7)* 2. Cells lining the acini contain small pyknotic nuclei and abundant bubbly cytoplasm *(Figs. 4.13.6 and 4.13.7)* 3. The nuclei are frequently apically located *(Fig. 4.13.7)* 4. Presence of intracytoplasmic secretory material superficially creates a monotonous appearance; however, nuclei are variably shaped and placed, characteristic of a benign hyperplastic process *(Fig. 4.13.7)*
Special studies	ER expression routinely assessed to predict response to adjuvant endocrine therapy; multigene assay may predict which patients may be spared radiation	None
Genetic abnormalities	Unknown	None
Treatment	Excise to negative margins, ± radiation, ± antiestrogen therapy	None; excision unnecessary if detected in a core biopsy specimen
Clinical implication	Eventuates in invasive carcinoma in approximately 30% of cases if not completely excised; with complete excision; recurrence rate approximately 8%–10% without radiation	None

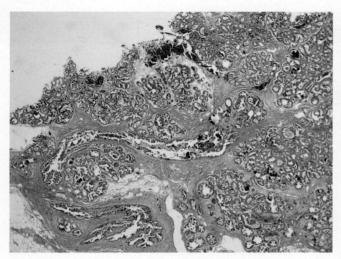

Figure 4.13.1   In this example of DCIS resembling hypersecretory hyperplasia, the low-power pattern shows an extensive and monotonous epithelial proliferation with numerous intraluminal projections in lobular units and true ducts.

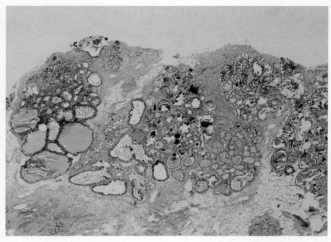

Figure 4.13.5   Hypersecretory hyperplasia is characterized by enlarged lobular units with variably dilated acini containing abundant secretory material associated with calcifications.

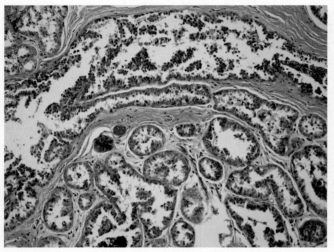

Figure 4.13.2   The malignant nuclei are multilayered and monotonous, forming numerous complex intraluminal papillary projections resembling hypersecretory hyperplasia.

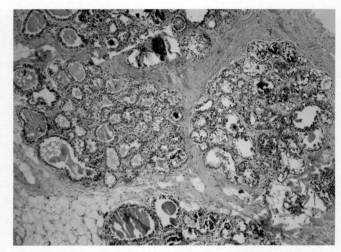

Figure 4.13.6   Cells lining the acini in hypersecretory hyperplasia contain small pyknotic nuclei and abundant bubbly cytoplasm.

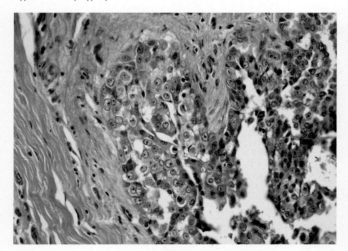

Figure 4.13.3   In this case, intermediate-grade nuclei with a uniform appearance and prominent nucleoli are diagnostic of DCIS.

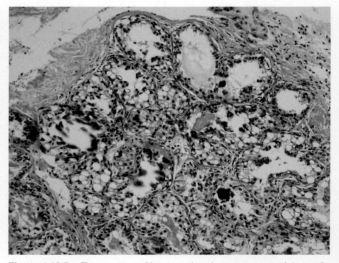

Figure 4.13.7   The presence of intracytoplasmic secretory material superficially creates a monotonous appearance; however, nuclei are variably shaped and placed, characteristic of a benign hyperplastic process. Note the nuclei are frequently apically located.

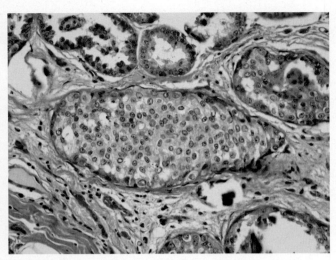

Figure 4.13.4   Focally the DCIS has a solid growth pattern.

	DCIS with a Pagetoid Growth Pattern	Radiation Change
Age	Adult women	Adult women
Location	Anywhere in the breast	Anywhere in the breast
Imaging findings	Architectural distortion, often linear or pleomorphic calcifications; may be associated with nipple discharge	Architectural distortion, occasionally calcifications
Etiology	Unknown	Radiation therapy for prior carcinoma (invasive or in situ)
Histology	1. Large ducts with cohesive clusters of neoplastic cells undermining the normal luminal epithelium *(Figs. 4.14.1–4.14.3)* 2. Nuclear uniformity and coarse chromatin patterns with prominent nucleoli *(Fig. 4.14.3)* 3. May form irregular and papillary projections into the duct lumen *(Fig. 4.14.3)* 4. Usually intermediate- or high-grade nuclei *(Figs. 4.14.3)*	1. Single layer or small clusters of enlarged luminal epithelial cells with large nuclei and ample amphophilic cytoplasm *(Figs. 4.14.4–4.14.6)* 2. Involves ducts and lobular units in radiation field and beyond 3. Cells frequently appear tethered to the epithelial lining by tendrils of cytoplasm; cytoplasm may appear foamy *(Fig. 4.14.5)* 4. Smudgy nuclear chromatin; occasional binucleate cells *(Fig. 4.14.5)* 5. Spaces otherwise lined by a normal luminal and myoepthelial component *(Figs. 4.14.4 and 4.14.5)* 6. Luminal calcifications may represent residual calcifications from eradicated DCIS, treatment-related fat necrosis, or calcified secretions unrelated to radiation therapy
Special studies	None to distinguish from radiation change; ER expression routinely assessed to predict response to adjuvant endocrine therapy; contamination with admixed normal luminal epithelial cells may alter results of multigene assays	None
Genetic Abnormalities	Unknown	None
Treatment	Excision to negative margins, ± radiation, ± antiestrogen therapy	None, excision is not indicated if detected in core biopsy specimen
Clinical implication	Growth pattern, often including patchy involvement of ducts, complicates margin assessment	None

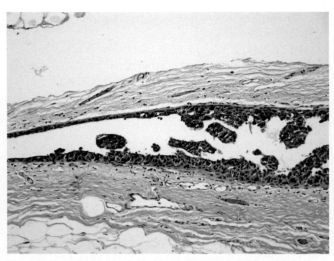

Figure 4.14.1 In this example of Pagetoid DCIS, cohesive clusters of neoplastic cells undermine the normal luminal epithelium of a large duct.

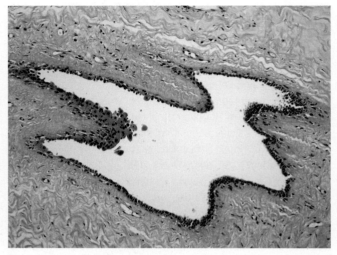

Figure 4.14.4 Radiation change: Scattered, enlarged luminal epithelial cells partially line this large duct.

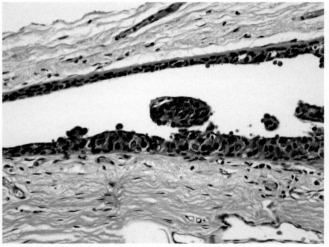

Figure 4.14.2 Pagetoid DCIS may form irregular and papillary-appearing projections into the duct lumen surmounted by an attenuated luminal epithelial layer.

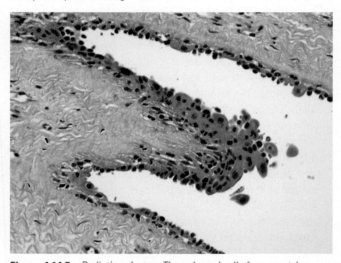

Figure 4.14.5 Radiation change: The enlarged cells form a patchy, single layer, have abundant amphophilic cytoplasm, and appear tethered to the epithelial lining. Occasional binucleate cells are present. Spaces otherwise lined by a normal luminal and myoepthelial component.

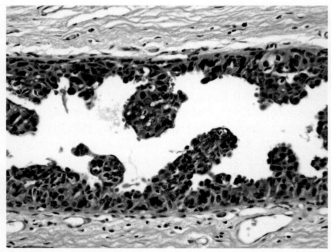

Figure 4.14.3 A Pagetoid pattern is most commonly seen in intermediate or high-grade DCIS characterized by nuclear irregularity, distinct chromatin patterns (coarse and open), and identifiable nucleoli.

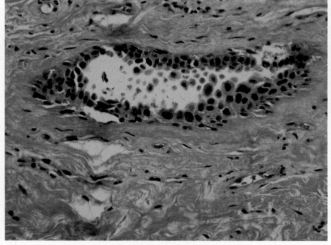

Figure 4.14.6 Tangential sectioning may create the appearance of multilayering. Foamy cytoplasm and smudgy chromatin with a viral cytopathic-like effect are characteristic of radiation change.

4 Ductal Carcinoma In Situ

SUGGESTED READINGS

Betsill WL Jr, Rosen PP, Lieberman PH, et al. Intraductal carcinoma. Long-term follow-up after treatment by biopsy alone. *JAMA.* 1978;239:1863–1867.

Bijker N, Meijnen P, Peterse JL, et al. Breast-conserving treatment with or without radiotherapy in ductal carcinoma-in-situ: ten-year results of European Organisation for Research and Treatment of Cancer randomized phase III trial 10853—a study by the EORTC Breast Cancer Cooperative Group and EORTC Radiotherapy Group. *J Clin Oncol.* 2006;24:3381–3387.

Caliskan M, Gatti G, Sosnovskikh I, et al. Paget's disease of the breast: the experience of the European Institute of Oncology and review of the literature. *Breast Cancer Res Treat.* 2008;112:513–521.

Carter D, Orr SL, Merino MJ. Intracystic papillary carcinoma of the breast. After mastectomy, radiotherapy or excisional biopsy alone. *Cancer.* 1983;52:14–19.

Chen YY, Hwang ES, Roy R, et al. Genetic and phenotypic characteristics of pleomorphic lobular carcinoma in situ of the breast. *Am J Surg Pathol.* 2009;33:1683–1694.

Collins IC, Tamimi, R., Baer, H., et al. Risk of invasive breast cancer in patients with ductal carcinoma in situ [DCIS] treated by diagnostic biopsy alone:results from the Nurses' Health Study. *Breast Cancer Res Treat.* 1994;88:1083.

Di Tommaso L, Franchi G, Destro A, et al. Toker cells of the breast. Morphological and immunohistochemical characterization of 40 cases. *Hum Pathol.* 2008;39:1295–1300.

Dupont WD, Page DL. Risk factors for breast cancer in women with proliferative breast disease. *N Engl J Med.* 1985;312:146–151.

Ernster VL, Barclay J, Kerlikowske K, et al. Incidence of and treatment for ductal carcinoma in situ of the breast. *JAMA* 1996;275:913–918.

Fisher ER, Costantino J, Fisher B, et al. Pathologic findings from the National Surgical Adjuvant Breast Project (NSABP) Protocol B-17. Five-year observations concerning lobular carcinoma in situ. *Cancer.* 1996;78:1403–1416.

Fisher ER, Dignam J, Tan-Chiu E, et al. Pathologic findings from the National Surgical Adjuvant Breast Project (NSABP) eight-year update of Protocol B-17: intraductal carcinoma. *Cancer.* 1999;86:429–438.

Fisher ER, Land SR, Fisher B, et al. Pathologic findings from the National Surgical Adjuvant Breast and Bowel Project: twelve-year observations concerning lobular carcinoma in situ. *Cancer.* 2004;100:238–244.

Foote F, Stewart, F. Lobular carcinoma in situ: a rare form of mammary carcinoma. *Am J Pathol.* 1941;17:491–496.

Hartmann LC, Sellers TA, Frost MH, et al. Benign breast disease and the risk of breast cancer. *N Engl J Med.* 2005;353:229–237.

Hilson JB, Schnitt SJ, Collins LC. Phenotypic alterations in myoepithelial cells associated with benign sclerosing lesions of the breast. *Am J Surg Pathol.* 2010;34:896–900.

Hughes LL, Wang M, Page DL, et al. Local excision alone without irradiation for ductal carcinoma in situ of the breast: a trial of the Eastern Cooperative Oncology Group. *J Clin Oncol.* 2009;27:5319–5324.

Jacobs TW, Pliss N, Kouria G, et al. Carcinomas in situ of the breast with indeterminate features: role of E-cadherin staining in categorization. *Am J Surg Pathol.* 2001;25:229–236.

Jensen R, Page DL. Epithelial hyperplasia. In: Elston CW, Ellis IO, eds. *The Breast.* 3rd ed. Edinburgh: Churchill Livingstone; 1998:65–89.

Lakhani SR, Ellis IO, Schnitt SJ, et al, eds. *WHO Classification of Tumors of the Breast.* 4 ed. Lyon: IARC; 2012.

Lester SC, Bose S, Chen YY, et al. Protocol for the examination of specimens from patients with ductal carcinoma in situ of the breast. *Arch Pathol Lab Med.* 2009;133:15–25.

Macdonald HR, Silverstein MJ, Lee LA, et al. Margin width as the sole determinant of local recurrence after breast conservation in patients with ductal carcinoma in situ of the breast. *Am J Surg.* 2006;192:420–422.

Maluf HM, Swanson PE, Koerner FC. Solid low-grade in situ carcinoma of the breast: role of associated lesions and E-cadherin in differential diagnosis. *Am J Surg Pathol.* 2001;25:237–244.

Marshall LM, Hunter DJ, Connolly JL, et al. Risk of breast cancer associated with atypical hyperplasia of lobular and ductal types. *Cancer Epidemiol Biomarkers Prev.* 1997;6:297–301.

Nassar H, Qureshi H, Adsay NV, et al. Clinicopathologic analysis of solid papillary carcinoma of the breast and associated invasive carcinomas. *Am J Surg Pathol.* 2006;30:501–507.

Otsuki Y, Yamada M, Shimizu S, et al. Solid-papillary carcinoma of the breast: clinicopathological study of 20 cases. *Pathol Int.* 2007;57:421–429.

Page DL, Dupont WD, Rogers LW, et al. Continued local recurrence of carcinoma 15–25 years after a diagnosis of low grade ductal carcinoma in situ of the breast treated only by biopsy. *Cancer.* 1995;76:1197–1200.

Page DL, Dupont WD, Rogers LW, et al. Intraductal carcinoma of the breast: follow-up after biopsy only. *Cancer.* 1982;49:751–758.

Page DL, Dupont WD, Rogers LW, et al. Atypical hyperplastic lesions of the female breast. A long-term follow-up study. *Cancer.* 1985;55:2698–2708.

Page DL, Kidd TE Jr, Dupont WD, et al. Lobular neoplasia of the breast: higher risk for subsequent invasive cancer predicted by more extensive disease. *Hum Pathol.* 1991;22:1232–1239.

Palacios J, Sarrio D, Garcia-Macias MC, et al. Frequent E-cadherin gene inactivation by loss of heterozygosity in pleomorphic lobular carcinoma of the breast. *Mod Pathol.* 2003;16:674–678.

Patchefsky AS, Schwartz GF, Finkelstein SD, et al. Heterogeneity of intraductal carcinoma of the breast. *Cancer.* 1989;63:731–741.

Pinder SE, Ellis IO, Schnitt SJ, et al. Microinvasive carcinoma. In: Lakhani SR, Ellis IO, Schnitt SJ, et al, eds. *WHO Classification of Tumors of the Breast.* Lyon: IARC; 2012:96–7.

Reis-Filho JS, Simpson PT, Jones C, et al. Pleomorphic lobular carcinoma of the breast: role of comprehensive molecular pathology in characterization of an entity. *J Pathol.* 2005;207:1–13.

Rosen PP, Kosloff C, Lieberman PH, et al. Lobular carcinoma in situ of the breast. Detailed analysis of 99 patients with average follow-up of 24 years. *Am J Surg Pathol.* 1978;2:225–251.

Sanders ME, Schuyler PA, Dupont WD, et al. The natural history of low-grade ductal carcinoma in situ of the breast in women treated by biopsy only revealed over 30 years of long-term follow-up. *Cancer.* 2005;103:2481–2484.

Sapino A, Frigerio A, Peterse JL, et al. Mammographically detected in situ lobular carcinomas of the breast. *Virchows Arch.* 2000;436:421–430.

Schwartz GF, Patchefsky AS, Finklestein SD, et al. Nonpalpable in situ ductal carcinoma of the breast. Predictors of multicentricity and microinvasion and implications for treatment. *Arch Surg.* 1989;124:29–32.

Shaaban AM, Sloane JP, West CR, et al. Histopathologic types of benign breast lesions and the risk of breast cancer: case–control study. *Am J Surg Pathol.* 2002;26:421–430.

Silverstein MJ, Lagios MD, Groshen S, et al. The influence of margin width on local control of ductal carcinoma in situ of the breast. *N Engl J Med.* 1999;340:1455–1461.

Sneige N, Wang J, Baker BA, et al. Clinical, histopathologic, and biologic features of pleomorphic lobular (ductal-lobular) carcinoma in situ of the breast: a report of 24 cases. *Mod Pathol.* 2002;15:1044–1050.

Solin LJ, Gray R, Baehner FL, et al. A multigene expression assay to predict local recurrence risk for ductal carcinoma in situ of the breast. *J Natl Cancer Inst.* 2013;105:701–710.

Tavassoli FA, Norris HJ. A comparison of the results of long-term follow-up for atypical intraductal hyperplasia and intraductal hyperplasia of the breast. *Cancer.* 1990;65:518–529.

Wheeler JE, Enterline HT, Roseman JM, et al. Lobular carcinoma in situ of the breast. Long-term followup. *Cancer.* 1974;34:554–563.

4 Ductal Carcinoma In Situ

5

Papillary and Sclerosing Lesions

	Sclerosed Papilloma	Fibroadenoma
Age	Adult women	Adult women, often bimodal distribution
Location	Often central, subareolar	Any location in breast
Imaging findings	Nodule or calcifications	Nodule or calcifications (in older women)
Etiology	Unknown	Unknown
Histology	1. Sclerotic nodule, usually retains a portion of duct wall lining *(Figs 5.1.1–5.1.4)* 2. Encysting fibrous duct wall contains entrapped epithelial elements that generally have a parallel arrangement *(Figs. 5.1.3 and 5.1.4)* 3. Peripheral epithelium often shows florid hyperplasia *(Figs. 5.1.3 and 5.1.4)* 4. Sclerosis may obliterate ductal lining epithelium *(Fig. 5.1.5)* 5. Central sclerosis entraps epithelial elements mimicking invasion *(Fig. 5.1.5)*, but parallel arrangement and maintenance of a dual cell population assure a benign diagnosis *(Fig. 5.1.6)*	1. Circumscribed proliferation of epithelium and stroma *(Figs. 5.1.7 and 5.1.8)* 2. Epithelium is evenly distributed within a paucicellular and myxoid stroma *(Figs. 5.1.9 and 5.1.10)* 3. Glandular epithelium is surrounded by (pericanalicular pattern) or compressed into cords (intracanallicular pattern) by the stromal proliferation *(Figs. 5.1.10 and 5.1.11)*, but no duct wall is present
Special studies	None to distinguish from fibroadenoma	None
Treatment	Excision is the usual recommendation for papillary lesions if diagnosed on core biopsy	Excision is not necessary, but is often performed for cosmesis; small fibroadenomas may be completely removed by core biopsy.
Clinical implication	Slightly increased risk of later cancer development (1.5×); risk is bilateral, but of insufficient magnitude to affect patient management	Women who have been diagnosed with a fibroadenoma are prone to develop additional fibroadenomas; however, women with fibroadenomas are not at increased risk for development of subsequent invasive carcinoma

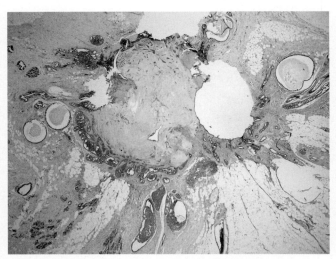

Figure 5.1.1   This sclerosed intraductal papilloma contains a central sclerotic nodule which deforms the adjacent epithelium.

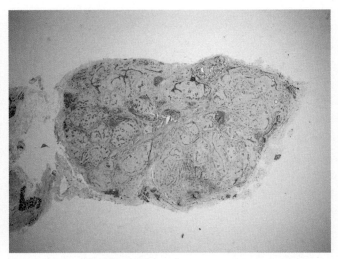

Figure 5.1.7   A fibroadenoma showing sharp circumscription and an abrupt interface with adjacent breast tissue.

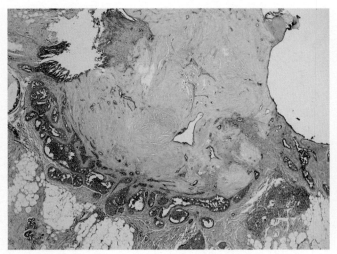

Figure 5.1.2   Central sclerosis entraps the epithelium and deforms areas of hyperplasia peripherally in this intraductal papilloma.

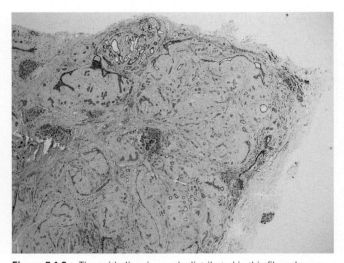

Figure 5.1.8   The epithelium is evenly distributed in this fibroadenoma.

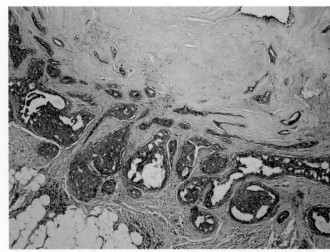

Figure 5.1.3   The entrapped glandular structures within this sclerosed papilloma generally maintain a parallel relationship. The peripheral epithelium shows hyperplasia without atypia.

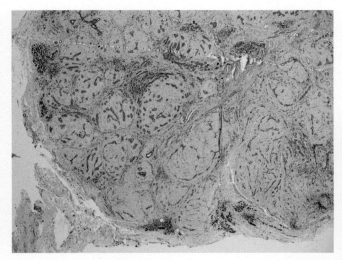

Figure 5.1.9   The bosselated edge and evenly distributed small glandular structures are characteristic of fibroadenoma.

5 Papillary/Sclerosing

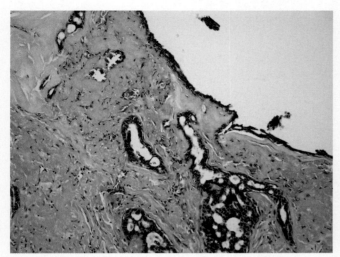

Figure 5.1.4 Focally a residual duct wall lining is present in this sclerosed intraductal papilloma (upper right).

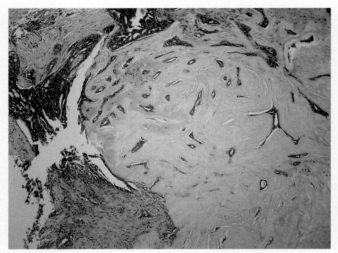

Figure 5.1.5 Sclerotic intraductal papilloma with entrapped glandular elements mimicking the pericanalicular pattern of a fibroadenoma. Note the previous biopsy site (lower left).

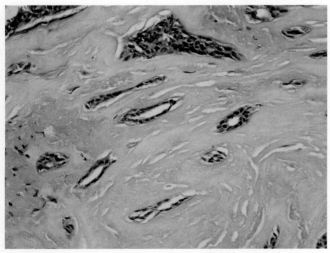

Figure 5.1.6 Entrapped glands in this sclerosed intraductal papilloma are distorted, but have a parallel arrangement and maintain a dual cell population.

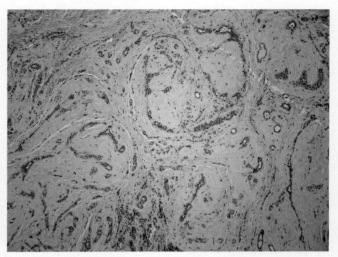

Figure 5.1.10 Several small nodular proliferations demonstrate a pericanalicular growth pattern in this fibroadenoma.

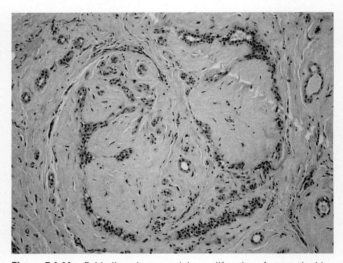

Figure 5.1.11 Epithelium rings a nodular proliferation of stroma in this fibroadenoma.

	Clustered Micropapillomas	Nipple Duct Adenoma
Age	Adult women	Adult women
Location	Often central, subareolar	Central, subareolar
Imaging finding	Calcifications or nodule	Superficial subareolar circumscribed nodule
Etiology	Unknown	Unknown
Histology	1. Lobulocentric epithelial proliferation *(Figs. 5.2.1 and 5.2.2)* 2. Solid proliferation of epithelium with slit-like peripheral secondary spaces *(Figs. 5.2.2 and 5.2.3)* 3. Residual fibrovascular cores may be subtle *(Fig. 5.2.4)*	1. Affects subareolar nipple ducts beneath the skin surface *(Figs. 5.2.5–5.2.7)* 2. Circumscribed, nodular epithelial proliferation *(Fig. 5.2.5)* with peripheral slit-like spaces 3. Frequently contains florid hyperplasia without atypia *(Figs. 5.2.6 and 5.2.7)*, characterized by irregular cell placement and indistinct cell borders
Special studies	None to distinguish from nipple adenoma	None
Treatment	Excision is not necessary for micropapillomas diagnosed on core biopsy	Excision with negative margins. May recur if incompletely excised.
Clinical implication	Slightly increased risk of later cancer development (1.5×); risk is bilateral, but of insufficient magnitude to affect patient management	When florid hyperplasia is a component, there is a slight increased risk of later cancer development (1.5×), similar to other proliferative lesions without atypia; risk is bilateral, but of insufficient magnitude to affect patient management

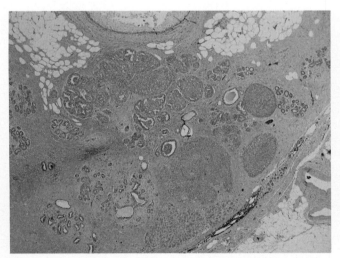

Figure 5.2.1 Clustered micropapillomas containing florid hyperplasia: Several lobular units and terminal ducts are expanded by an epithelial proliferation.

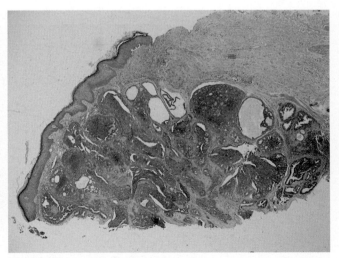

Figure 5.2.5 Nipple duct adenoma consists of a nodular proliferation of epithelium involving nipple ducts just beneath the skin.

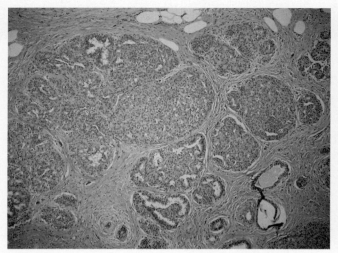

Figure 5.2.2   A lobulocentric configuration is maintained despite distortion of these clustered micropapillomas by hyperplasia.

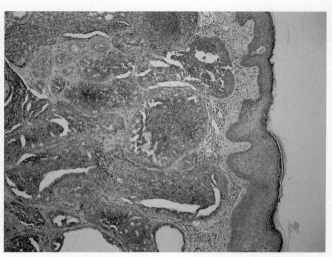

Figure 5.2.6   The nipple ducts contain an exuberant epithelial proliferation with numerous slit-like spaces characteristic of florid hyperplasia without atypia.

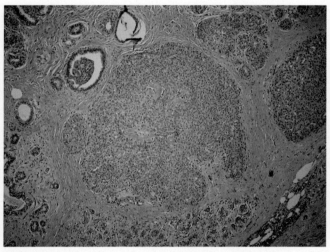

Figure 5.2.3   The fibrovascular cores of these clustered micropapillomas are almost obliterated by florid hyperplasia without atypia.

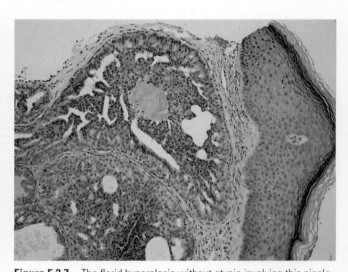

Figure 5.2.7   The florid hyperplasia without atypia involving this nipple duct adenoma has slit-like peripheral secondary spaces and the cell placement is irregular. Focal punctate necrosis is common in this setting.

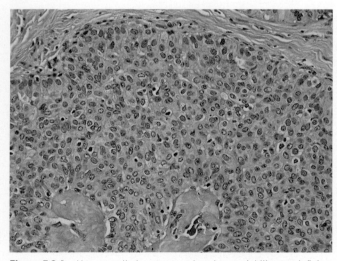

Figure 5.2.4   Uneven cell placement and nuclear variability are defining of florid hyperplasia involving a micropapilloma. Note the sclerosed fibrovascular cores (bottom).

	Sclerosed papilloma	Adenomyoepithelioma
Age	Adult women	Adult women
Location	Retroareolar (solitary) or peripheral (may be multiple)	Retroareolar, usually solitary
Imaging findings	Nodular density, duct filling defect on galactogram	Nodular density
Etiology	Unknown	Unknown
Histology	1. Dilated duct containing arborizing fibrovascular cores subtended by epithelium *(Figs. 5.3.1–5.3.3)* 2. Glandular structures consist of luminal epithelial and myoepithelial cells *(Fig. 5.3.4)* 3. The glandular structures are separated from each other by stroma *(Figs 5.3.4–5.3.6)* 4. Myoepithelial cells may be prominent, but do not present a solid growth pattern *(Figs. 5.3.4–5.3.6)*	1. Round to ovoid, often lobulated nodule, more solid than the typical papilloma and may be partially surrounded by a fibrotic duct wall *(Figs. 5.3.7–5.3.9)* 2. Bland myoepithelial cells *(Fig. 5.3.10)* forming solid sheets *(Fig. 5.3.11)* are a prominent component 3. Numerous small glandular structures, many with obliterated lumens resemble sclerosing adenosis *(Figs. 5.3.12 and 5.3.13)*
Special studies	Immunohistochemistry using antibodies to myoepithelial markers demonstrates a normally distributed (basal) myoepithelial component	Immunohistochemistry using antibodies to myoepithelial markers such as p63 demonstrates a prominent (usually more than half of the lesion) myoepithelial component *(Fig. 5.3.14)* while CK5/6 is less specific and variably expressed by both the epithelial and myoepithelial components *(Fig. 5.3.15)*
Treatment	Excision is the usual recommendation for papillary lesions	Conservative excision to negative margins to avoid local recurrence; rare recurrences may be associated with low-grade adenosquamous carcinoma or spindle cell metaplastic carcinoma
Clinical implication	Slightly increased risk of later cancer development for intraductal papilloma (1.5×); risk is bilateral, but of insufficient magnitude to affect patient management. If atypical ductal hyperplasia (ADH) or ductal carcinoma in situ (DCIS) is present, subsequent risk is greater and ipsilateral (see example 5.5).	Benign lesion with capacity for local recurrence. Lesions reported to be associated with malignant behavior were also accompanied by coexistent DCIS or metaplastic carcinoma. In the absence of DCIS or metaplastic carcinoma, adenomyoepthelioma is a benign entity.

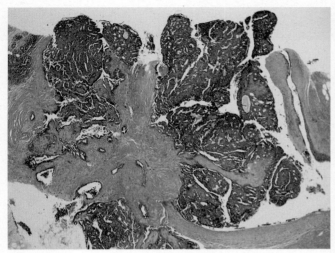

Figure 5.3.1   Intraductal papilloma: The encysting fibrous duct wall surrounds arborizing fibrovascular cores, lined by proliferating epithelium; central sclerosis contains entrapped glands.

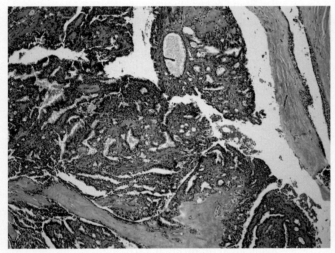

Figure 5.3.2   A sclerosed intraductal papilloma with maintenance of arborizing fibrovascular cores. Only a small portion of the duct lumen with lining remains (far right).

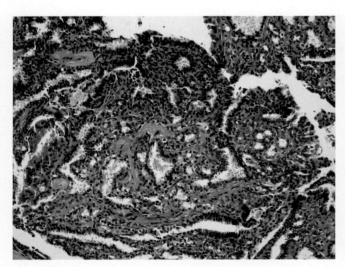

Figure 5.3.3   Small glandular structures are separated by intervening stroma. Focally the epithelium has apocrine cytology.

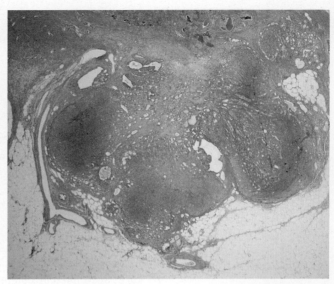

Figure 5.3.7   Adenomyoepithelioma with a characteristic lobulated and solid appearance at low magnification.

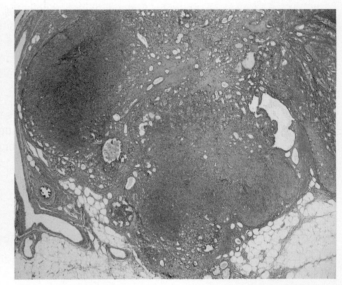

Figure 5.3.8   The epithelial proliferation in adenomyoepithelioma is predominantly solid, with an encysting fibrous rind, a remnant of a former duct wall.

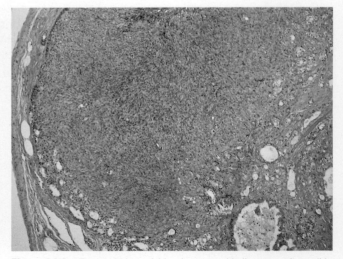

Figure 5.3.9   The lobulations of this adenomyoepithelioma contain a solid, spindle cell proliferation centrally and glandular elements at the periphery.

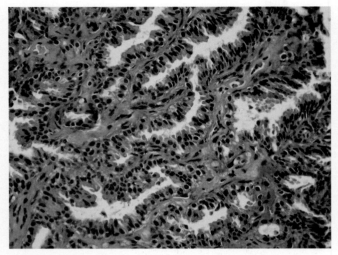

Figure 5.3.4 Glandular structures contain luminal epithelial and myo-epithelial cells.

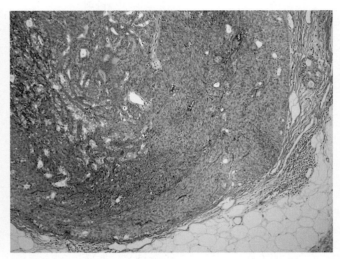

Figure 5.3.10 Glandular elements are intermixed with the solid, spindled proliferation in this adenomyoepithelioma.

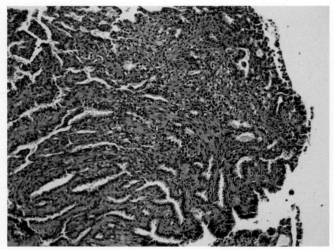

Figure 5.3.5 The epithelium of the papilloma shows a mixture of epi-thelial and myoepithelial cells.

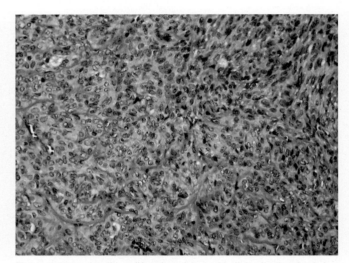

Figure 5.3.11 A solid proliferation of myoepithelial cells showing spin-dled but varied nuclei that are overlapping in this adenomyoepithelioma.

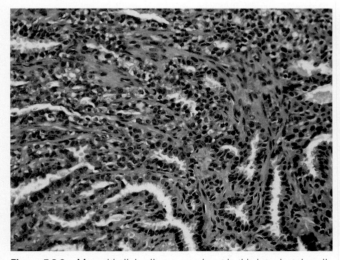

Figure 5.3.6 Myoepithelial cells are prominent in this intraductal papil-loma, but foci of solid growth are absent.

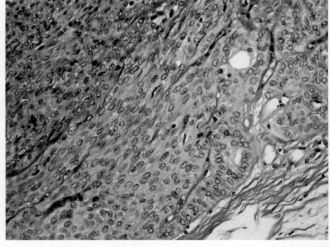

Figure 5.3.12 The proliferating myoepithelial cells have spindled nuclei and clear cytoplasm in this adenomyoepithelioma. Note adjacent glandu-lar differentiation.

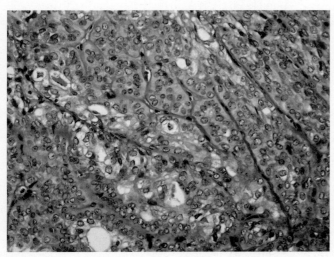

Figure 5.3.13   Adenomyoepithelioma showing an area of glandular differentiation. Nuclear variability and overlap are characteristic.

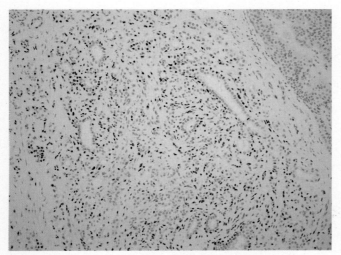

Figure 5.3.14   Immunohistochemical expression of nuclear p63 by the myoepithelial component of an adenomyoepithelioma

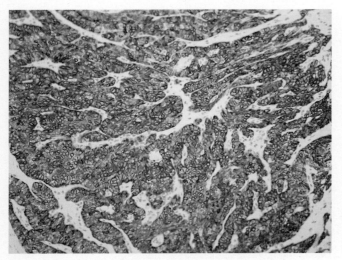

Figure 5.3.15   Immunohistochemical expression of high molecular weight cytokeratin (CK5/6) by the spindled myoepithelial proliferation in adenomyoepithelioma.

	Sclerosed Adenotic Papilloma	Nodular Sclerosing Adenosis
Age	Adult women	Adult women
Location	Often central, subareolar	May occur anywhere in the breast
Imaging findings	Calcifications or nodule	Calcifications, may be mass forming (nodular adenosis or adenosis tumor)
Etiology	Unknown	Unknown
Histology	1. Rounded nodule of small glandular structures, encased by a dense fibrous rind *(Figs. 5.4.1 and 5.4.2)* 2. A small amount of duct lining may remain *(Fig. 5.4.1)* 3. Central sclerosis entraps epithelial elements *(Figs. 5.4.1 and 5.4.3)* 4. An encysting fibrous duct wall contains entrapped epithelial elements that generally have a parallel arrangement *(Figs. 5.4.2 and 5.4.3)* 5. Glandular elements are compressed by sclerosis but myoepithelial cells are maintained *(Figs. 5.4.4 and 5.4.5)*	1. Several lobular units involved by sclerosing adenosis coalesce to form a lobulated mass (nodular adenosis), but a lobulocentric configuration is maintained *(Fig. 5.4.6)* 2. Individual lobular units contain numerous small acini, which retain myoepithelial and luminal layers *(Fig 5.4.7)* 3. Acini are frequently distorted and compressed, losing their lumens, especially at the periphery of the lesion *(Figs. 5.4.8–5.4.10)* 4. Myoepithelial cells may compose the majority of the lesion when sclerosis is prominent *(Figs. 5.4.8 and 5.4.10)*
Special studies	None to distinguish from sclerosing adenosis	None to distinguish from sclerosed intraductal papilloma; immunohistochemical studies using antibodies to myoepithelial markers such as p63 may be helpful in recognizing benignancy
Treatment	Excision is the usual recommendation for papillary lesions	Excision unnecessary if detected on core needle biopsy with concordant imaging studies
Clinical implication	Slightly increased risk of later cancer development (1.5×); risk is bilateral, but of insufficient magnitude to affect patient management	Slightly increased risk of later cancer development (1.5×); risk is bilateral, but of insufficient magnitude to affect patient management

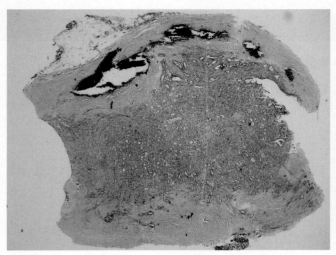

Figure 5.4.1   Sclerotic, adenotic intraductal papilloma characterized by a nodular configuration of small glandular structures surrounded by a dense fibrous, partially calcified wall. The duct lumen is essentially obliterated in this example.

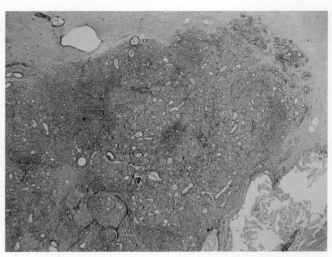

Figure 5.4.6   Nodular sclerosing adenosis consisting of a lobulated mass of small glandular structures formed by the aggregation of individual lobular units involved by sclerosing adenosis.

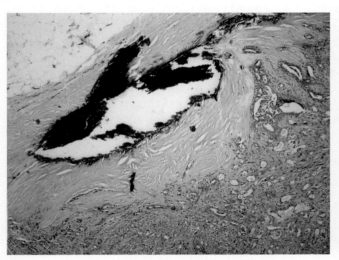

Figure 5.4.2   Predominantly smooth contour of small glandular structures adjacent to the encysting fibrous duct wall in a sclerotic, adenotic intraductal papilloma.

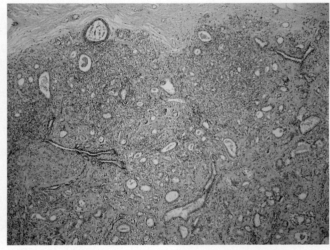

Figure 5.4.7   The proliferation of small glands and myoepithelial cells is not associated with a fibrous duct wall in nodular sclerosing adenosis.

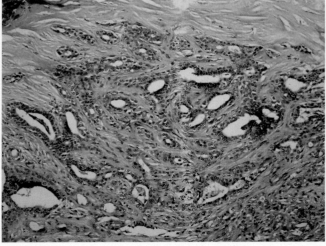

Figure 5.4.3   Sclerotic, adenotic intraductal papilloma: At the periphery of the nodular proliferation, the glandular structures are often parallel to each other.

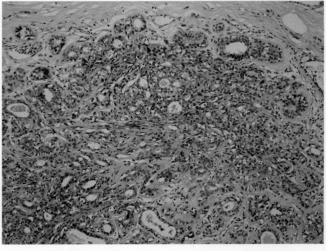

Figure 5.4.8   Many of the epithelial structures of nodular sclerosing adenosis are compressed without recognizable lumens.

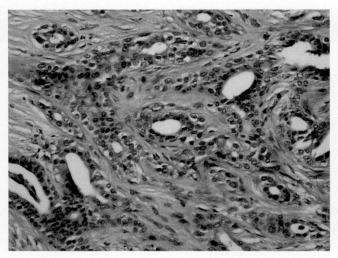

Figure 5.4.4 A myoepithelial layer is evident in the entrapped glandular structures in this sclerotic, adenotic intraductal papilloma.

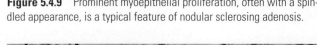

Figure 5.4.9 Prominent myoepithelial proliferation, often with a spindled appearance, is a typical feature of nodular sclerosing adenosis.

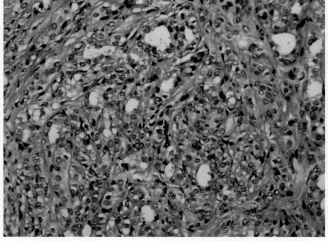

Figure 5.4.5 In many areas of this sclerotic, adenotic intraductal papilloma, few glandular lumens remain.

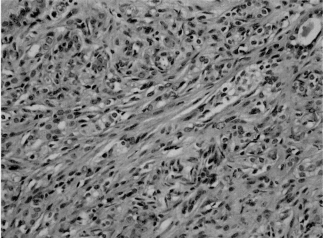

Figure 5.4.10 Nodular sclerosing adenosis: The presence of clear cytoplasm is characteristic of myoepithelial cells.

5 Papillary/Sclerosing

	ADH in Papilloma	Usual Hyperplasia in a Papilloma
Age	Adult women	Adult women, rarely adolescents
Location	Larger papillomas are typically central (retroareolar) while smaller or multiple papillomas are peripheral	Anywhere in the breast
Imaging findings	Nodular density, rarely associated calcifications, internal vascularity	Nodular density, rarely associated calcifications, internal vascularity
Etiology	Unknown	Unknown
Histology	1. Proliferation of uniform cells with low-grade nuclei associated with fibrovascular cores *(Fig. 5.5.1)* 2. Evenly placed cells, well-defined intercellular cell borders, cribriform or solid pattern most common *(Figs. 5.5.2 and 5.5.3)* 3. Extent of contiguous involvement less than 3 mm *(Figs. 5.5.3 and 5.3.4)*	1. Intraductal epithelial proliferation supported by fibrovascular cores *(Figs. 5.5.5 and 5.5.6)* 2. Cells show overlap and irregular placement *(Figs. 5.5.7 and 5.5.8)* 3. Indistinct cell borders and variably shaped nuclei *(Figs. 5.5.7 and 5.5.8)* 4. Secondary spaces are irregular and slit-like, located peripherally *(Fig. 5.5.7)* 5. Heliotrope inclusions common
Special studies	Immunohistochemical analysis may show single basally located, frequently patchy, p63-positive myoepithelial cells; loss of CK5/6 expression characteristic but not defining	None; variable expression of CK5/6
Treatment	Excision if detected on core biopsy	Conservative excision if papilloma diagnosed in core biopsy to exclude atypical hyperplasia in unsampled papilloma
Clinical implication	Increased risk for later cancer development in ipsilateral breast; differs from bilateral risk associated with ADH involving nonpapillomatous breast tissue	Slightly increased risk of later cancer development (1.5×); risk is bilateral, but of insufficient magnitude to affect patient management

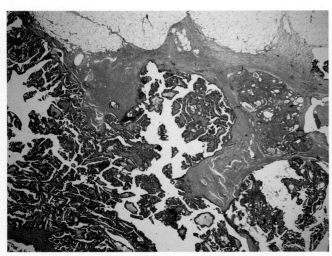

Figure 5.5.1 Intraductal papilloma containing ADH (upper right): Fibrovascular cores are surmounted by a proliferation of uniform cells with solid and cribriform architecture.

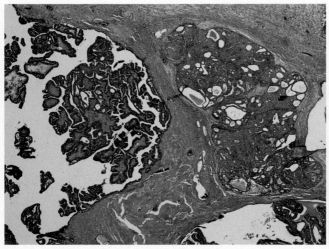

Figure 5.5.2 A localized solid and cribriform proliferation of epithelial cells is characteristic of ADH within an intraductal papilloma.

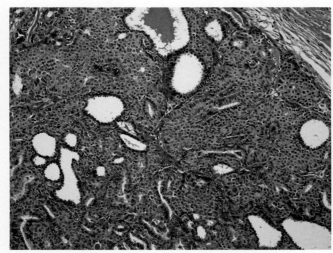

Figure 5.5.3 Cells are uniform and evenly placed, but occupy less than 3 mm in contiguous growth, defining ADH within an intraductal papilloma.

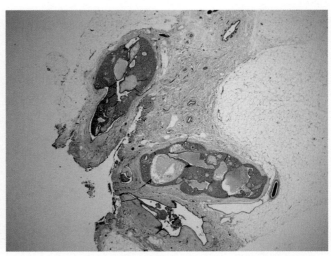

Figure 5.5.5 The predominantly solid epithelial proliferation in this intraductal papilloma surmounts large, sclerotic fibrovascular cores.

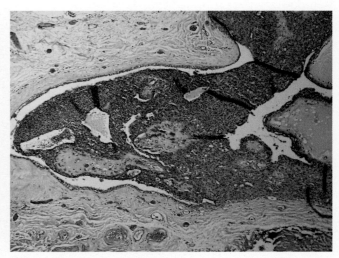

Figure 5.5.6 In this intraductal papilloma, solid-pattern florid hyperplasia distends the duct, although much of the ductal lining is still evident. Note the prominent fibrovascular cores.

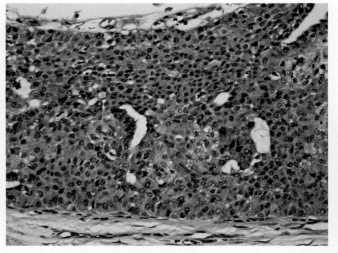

Figure 5.5.7 Although the epithelial proliferation is exuberant in this intraductal papilloma, nuclear variability and overlap assure a benign diagnosis of florid hyperplasia.

5 Papillary/Sclerosing

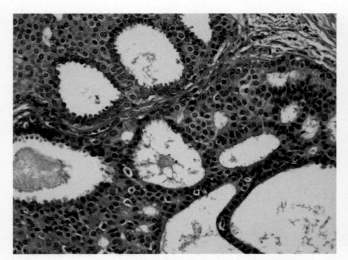

Figure 5.5.4 Distinct cell borders, cellular uniformity, and even cell placement are features of ADH involving an intraductal papilloma.

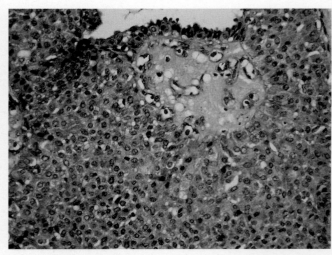

Figure 5.5.8 Indistinct cell borders, nuclear variability, and overlap are characteristic of florid hyperplasia without atypia involving an intraductal papilloma.

	ADH in Papilloma	DCIS Involving a Papilloma
Age	Adult women	Adult women
Location	Larger papillomas are typically central (retroareolar) while smaller or multiple papillomas are peripheral	Larger papillomas are typically central (retroareolar) while smaller papillomas are often peripheral and multiple
Imaging findings	Nodular density, rarely associated calcifications, internal vascularity	Density or nodule, rarely calcifications, may show internal vascularity
Etiology	Unknown	Unknown
Histology	1. Intraductal proliferation of uniform, evenly placed cells with low-grade nuclei associated with fibrovascular cores (Fig. 5.6.1) 2. Duct wall delimits the epithelial proliferation, which shows cribriform architecture (Fig. 5.6.2) 3. Uniform cells with well-defined cell borders; no focus larger than 3 mm (Figs. 5.6.3 and 5.6.4) 4. Residual normal epithelium is polarized at the periphery (Fig. 5.6.4)	1. Nodular proliferation of cells within a dilated duct (Fig. 5.6.5) 2. Cells are evenly placed, often with a cribriform or solid pattern (Fig. 5.6.6) 3. Extent of contiguous involvement is more than 3 mm, and generally at least 5 mm (Fig. 5.6.6) 4. Uniform cells form back to back cribriform structures, without intervening stroma (Figs. 5.5.7–5.6.9) 5. DCIS is often present in adjacent non-papillomatous ducts 6. Encysting fibrous wall may be densely sclerotic
Special studies	Immunohistochemical studies for myoepithelial markers show a single basally located, frequently patchy, myoepithelial layer; loss of CK5/6 expression is characteristic but should not be used to gauge the size of the lesion as loss may also be seen in non-atypical lesions	Some retention of myoepithelial cells by immunohistochemistry; however, their absence does not equate to a diagnosis of invasive carcinoma
Treatment	Excision if detected on core biopsy	Breast conserving surgery ± radiation; mastectomy may be required for extensive disease; ± antiestrogen therapy
Clinical implication	Increased risk for later cancer development in ipsilateral breast; differs from bilateral risk associated with ADH involving nonpapillomatous breast tissue	Risk of local recurrence related to size of DCIS, grade, and margin status

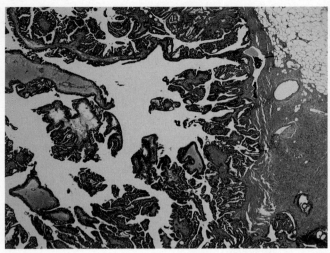

Figure 5.6.1   ADH in an intraductal papilloma. A densely fibrotic duct wall surrounds an epithelial proliferation associated with fibrovascular cores.

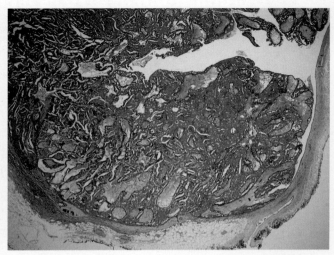

Figure 5.6.5   A fibrous duct wall and fibrovascular cores define this lesion as an intraductal papilloma. The presence of a solid and cribriform proliferation extending more than 5.0 mm requires a diagnosis of DCIS.

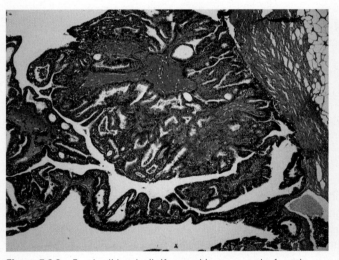

Figure 5.6.2   Focal solid and cribriform architecture results from the even cell placement characteristic of ADH.

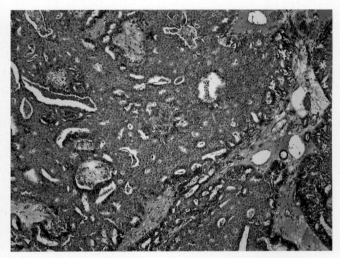

Figure 5.6.6   The solid and cribriform pattern of low-grade DCIS does not contain intervening stroma. This unsupported epithelial proliferation is diagnosed as low-grade DCIS, involving an intraductal papilloma.

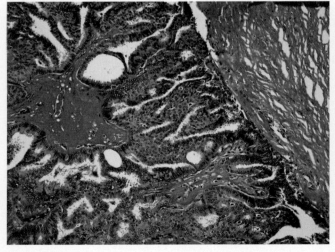

Figure 5.6.3   Intervening stroma is present between the monotonous cell proliferation of ADH in an intraductal papilloma.

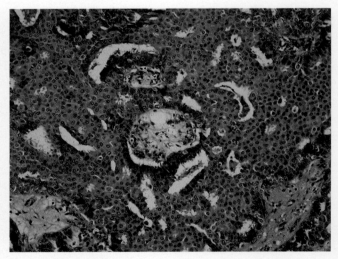

Figure 5.6.7   Back-to-back glands of DCIS involving an intraductal papilloma. Note the fibrovascular cores centrally.

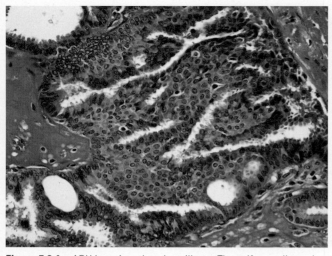

Figure 5.6.4   ADH in an intraductal papilloma. The uniform cell population is less than 3.0 mm in continuity; normally polarized cells remain.

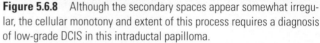

Figure 5.6.8   Although the secondary spaces appear somewhat irregular, the cellular monotony and extent of this process requires a diagnosis of low-grade DCIS in this intraductal papilloma.

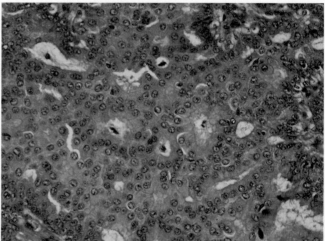

Figure 5.6.9   The solid growth pattern shows microrosette formation in low-grade DCIS involving an intraductal papilloma.

	DCIS Involving Multiple Papillomas	Encysted Noninvasive Papillary Carcinoma
Age	Adult women	Adult women, often elderly
Location	Anywhere in the breast	Subareolar or central breast
Imaging findings	Architectural distortion, may contain pleomorphic or linear calcifications	Nodular mass, may appear cystic and solid, may have internal vascularity
Etiology	Unknown	Unknown
Histology	1. Involvement of multiple intraductal and/or micropapillomas and adjacent ducts by DCIS *(Figs. 5.7.1–5.7.3)* 2. DCIS is often extensive 3. Pure micropapillary pattern or mixed micropapillary and cribriform patterns, most common *(Figs. 5.7.4–5.7.6)* 4. DCIS in adjacent ducts may have more rigid architecture; however, the cytologic features are the same as the DCIS within the papilloma *(Fig. 5.7.7)* 5. May be difficult to diagnose on core biopsy as skip areas common and extent may not be evident until definitive excision	1. Large intraductal papilloma with a thick layer of encysting fibrous tissue which obliterates the duct wall *(Fig. 5.7.8)* 2. The papilloma is replaced or nearly replaced by confluent DCIS characterized by a uniform cell population *(Fig. 5.7.9)* 3. DCIS is confined to the papilloma with limited involvement of immediately adjacent ducts *(Fig. 5.7.8)* 4. Proliferating epithelium is associated with small fibrovascular cores *(Fig. 5.7.10)* 5. DCIS may be of any grade but is usually low or intermediate *(Figs. 5.7.10 and 5.7.11)* 6. DCIS may be of any pattern, most commonly cribriform, solid or micropapillary *(Fig 5.7.11)*
Special studies	None; lack of CK5/6 expression only in low-grade DCIS	None routinely used; loss of CK5/6 expression may support the diagnosis in some low-grade cases but should not be used to establish the diagnosis; absence of myoepithelial cell markers should not be equated as invasive
Treatment	Breast conservation ± radiation; vs. mastectomy for extensive disease; ± antiestrogen therapy	Excision to negative margins, radiation therapy may not be required
Clinical implication	Risk of local recurrence related to size of DCIS, grade, and margin distance; frequently more extensive than other forms of DCIS and may require mastectomy for eradication	Long term follow-up studies have shown clinical behavior of these lesions is that of DCIS; American Joint Committee on Cancer (AJCC) and College of American Pathologists (CAP) guidelines stage these as DCIS

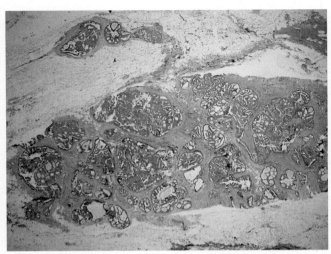

Figure 5.7.1   Low-grade DCIS involving multiple papillomas: Cribriform and micropapillary architecture expands the involved spaces.

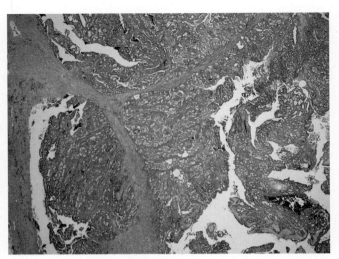

Figure 5.7.8   Encysted noninvasive papillary carcinoma: A single duct is greatly expanded by a neoplastic proliferation. Although a duct lining is no longer evident, the encysting fibrous tissue is characteristic of a duct wall, supporting a diagnosis of in situ carcinoma.

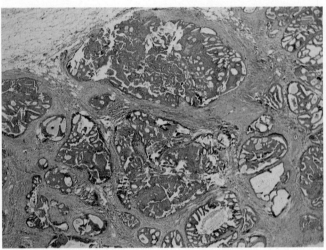

Figure 5.7.2   Clustered micropapillomas and adjacent ducts contain a uniform cell population characteristic of low-grade DCIS.

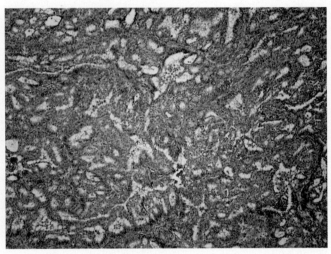

Figure 5.7.9   Small fibrovascular cores are associated with a pronounced proliferation of epithelium forming solid and cribriform structures in encysted, noninvasive papillary carcinoma.

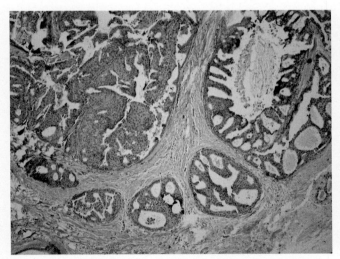

Figure 5.7.3   DCIS adjacent to and involving micropapillomas, showing cribriform and micropapillary architecture.

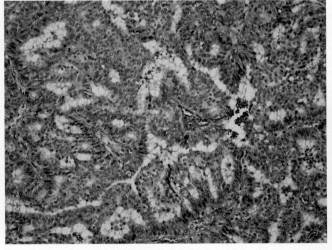

Figure 5.7.10   Encysted, noninvasive papillary carcinoma: An epithelial proliferation forms small glandular structures that are arranged "back-to-back," without intervening stroma.

5 Papillary/Sclerosing

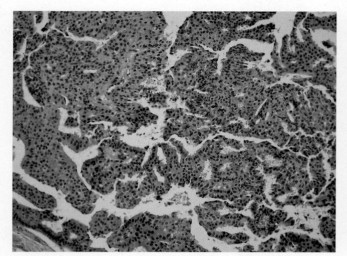

Figure 5.7.4   Arborizing fibrovascular fronds are surrounded by solid and cribriform architecture in this example of low-grade DCIS within a papilloma

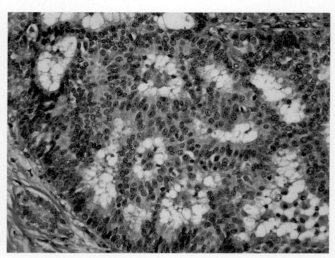

Figure 5.7.11   Solid and cribriform areas as well as low-grade nuclei are characteristic of encysted, noninvasive papillary carcinoma.

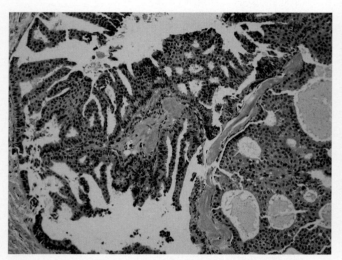

Figure 5.7.5   Cribriform and micropapillay patterns of DCIS within a papilloma.

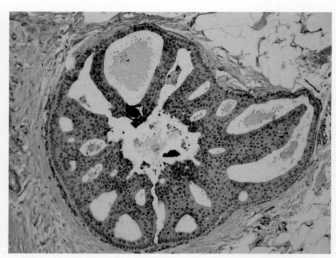

Figure 5.7.7   DCIS involving a duct adjacent to the papilloma. Low-grade nuclei and cribriform architecture are common in this presentation.

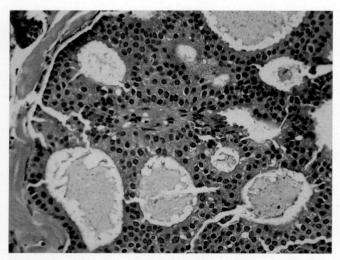

Figure 5.7.6   Low-grade DCIS involving a micropapilloma. A subtle fibrovascular core is surrounded by a proliferation of uniform cells arranged in a cribriform architecture.

	Sclerosing Adenosis	Radial Scar
Age	Adult women	Adult women
Location	Anywhere in the breast	Anywhere in the breast
Imaging findings	Calcifications, may be mass-forming (nodular sclerosing adenosis)	Spiculated mass, may contain calcification; architectural distortion
Etiology	Unknown	Unknown
Histology	1. Lobulocentric process containing a proliferation of small acini which maintain their myoepithelial and luminal layers *(Figs. 5.8.1 and 5.8.2)* 2. The acini are frequently distorted and compressed, losing their lumina *(Fig. 5.8.3)* 3. In lesions with marked sclerosis, myoepithelial cells may compose the majority of the lesion *(Fig. 5.8.4)* 4. Sclerosis predominates centrally, while some glandular structures are usually preserved peripherally but they may be flattened, forming a blunted or microlobulated interface with the surrounding mammary parenchyma *(Figs. 5.8.2 and 5.8.5)* 5. Several involved lobular units may coalesce to form a lobulated mass (nodular sclerosing adenosis), which maintains a lobulocentric configuration *(Fig. 5.8.2)* 6. The presence of sclerosing adenosis should prompt a careful search for atypical lobular hyperplasia, because of their frequent coexistence	1. Region of central elastosis and sclerosis from which epithelial elements radiate *(Fig. 5.8.6)* 2. Round and angulated glandular structures are frequently entrapped and distorted within the central region *(Figs. 5.8.8–5.8.10)* 3. Epithelial elements typically consist of usual hyperplasia, sclerosing adenosis, and micropapillomas *(Fig. 5.8.8)* 4. Glandular structures are confined to the radial sclerosis without infiltration into adipose tissue *(Fig. 5.8.7)* 5. Glandular structures have a luminal epithelial layer and a less conspicuous myoepithelial layer which may be compressed and have pyknotic nuclei *(Figs. 5.8.8–5.8.10)*
Special studies	No special studies to distinguish from radial scar; myoepithelial markers such as p63 may be helpful in recognizing benignancy	None to separate from sclerosing adenosis; immnuohistochemistry for myoepithelial markers highlights an intact (but frequently patchy) myoepithelial layer. Diagnosis is based predominantly on H&E morphology, because myoepithelial marker expression may be reduced in benign sclerosing lesions.
Treatment	Excision unnecessary if detected on core biopsy with concordant imaging	Radial scars are frequently excised based on mammographic concern; in the absence of atypical hyperplasia on core biopsy, there is no evidence to support this practice
Clinical implication	Slightly increased risk of later cancer development (1.5×); risk is bilateral, but of insufficient magnitude to affect patient management	Subsequent carcinoma risk is that attributed to any epithelial proliferation that may be present within the radial scar, i.e., usual hyperplasia or atypical hyperplasia

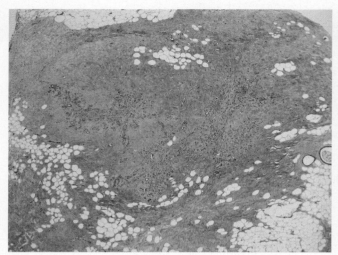

Figure 5.8.1   Several involved lobular units may coalesce to form a lobulated mass (nodular sclerosing adenosis), which maintains a lobulocentric configuration.

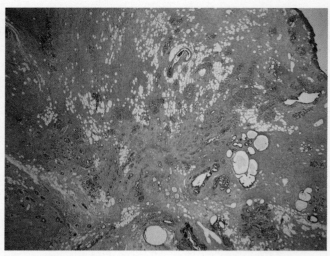

Figure 5.8.6   Radial scar showing central elastosis and sclerosis from which epithelial elements radiate.

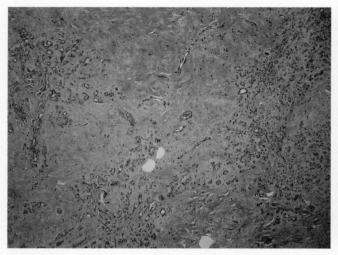

Figure 5.8.2   Intralobular specialized connective tissue is replaced by sclerosis, resulting in distortion and compression of acini in sclerosing adenosis.

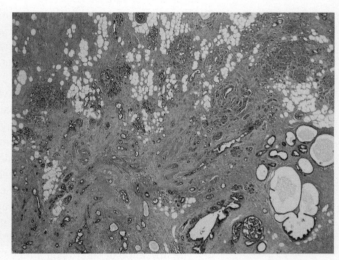

Figure 5.8.7   The glandular structures of a radial scar are present within the confines of the sclerosis, without infiltration into adipose tissue.

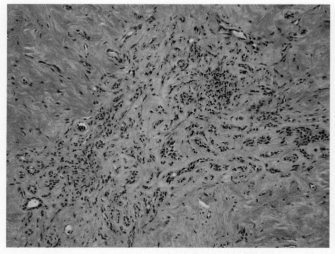

Figure 5.8.3   In lesions with marked sclerosis, myoepithelial cells may compose the majority of the cells in sclerosing adenosis. Peripherally, small glandular structures are present.

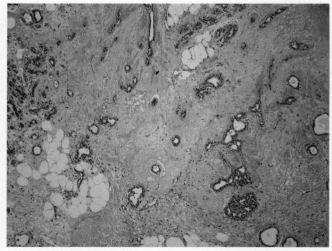

Figure 5.8.8   The periphery of a radial scar may contain usual hyperplasia, sclerosing adenosis, and micropapillomas.

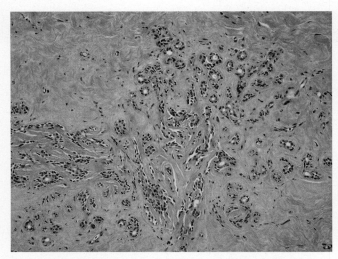

Figure 5.8.4   Sclerosing adenosis showing predominant sclerosis centrally with some preservation of glandular structures peripherally. The glands may be flattened, forming a blunted or microlobulated interface with the surrounding mammary parenchyma.

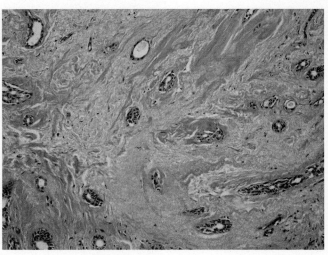

Figure 5.8.9   Round and angulated glandular structures are frequently entrapped and distorted within the central region of a radial scar.

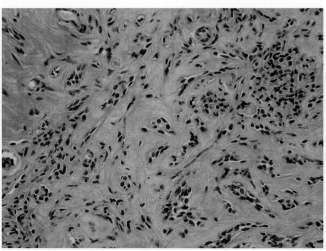

Figure 5.8.5   The intralobular specialized connective tissue is densely sclerotic but lacks elastosis.

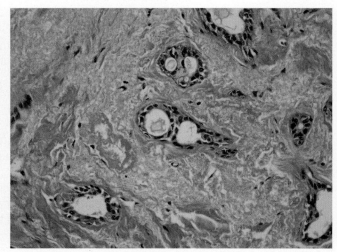

Figure 5.8.10   Central, entrapped glandular structures within a radial scar have a luminal epithelial layer and a less conspicuous myoepithelial layer with pyknotic nuclei which may be compressed.

	Sclerosing Adenosis	Microglandular Adenosis
Age	Adult women	Adult women, usually older than women with sclerosing adenosis
Location	Anywhere in the breast	Anywhere in the breast
Imaging findings	Calcifications, may be mass-forming (nodular sclerosing adenosis)	Often incidental finding, but may present as an irregular density or parenchymal distortion
Etiology	Unknown	Unknown
Histology	1. Lobulocentric process containing a proliferation of small acini which maintain their myoepithelial and luminal layers *(Figs. 5.9.1–5.9.6)* 2. The acini are frequently distorted and compressed, losing their lumina *(Figs. 5.9.4 and 5.9.6)* 3. In lesions with marked sclerosis, myoepithelial cells may compose the majority of the lesion *(Fig. 5.9.6)* 4. Sclerosis predominates centrally while some glandular structures are usually preserved peripherally but may be flattened, forming a blunted or microlobulated interface with the surrounding mammary parenchyma *(Fig. 5.9.2)* 5. The presence of sclerosing adenosis should prompt a careful search for atypical lobular hyperplasia because of their frequent association	1. Infiltrative, nonlobulocentric proliferation of uniform, small round glands within unspecialized connective tissue and fat *(Figs. 5.9.7 and 5.9.8)* 2. Regular round glands are not compressed by stroma and rarely show gland fusion *(Fig. 5.9.9)* 3. Glands are lined by a single layer of cuboidal epithelial cells with round nuclei and clear cytoplasm, lacking apical snouts *(Figs. 5.9.9 and 5.9.10)* 4. There is no cytologic atypia or mitotic activity *(Figs. 5.9.9 and 5.9.10)* 5. Scattered glands contain eosinophilic secretory material *(Fig. 5.9.10)* 6. Although surrounded by a basement membrane the glands lack a myoepithelial layer
Special studies	Myoepithelial marker expression retained	The glands demonstrate strong expression of S100 protein *(Fig. 5.9.11)* but are negative for expression of ER, PR, and p63
Treatment	Excision unnecessary if detected on core biopsy with concordant imaging	Excision unnecessary if incidental finding; if mass lesion, complete excision to negative margins
Clinical implication	Slightly increased risk of later cancer development (1.5×); risk is bilateral, but of insufficient magnitude to affect patient management	No metastatic capacity, although extensive lesions may require mastectomy because of a diffusely infiltrative growth pattern

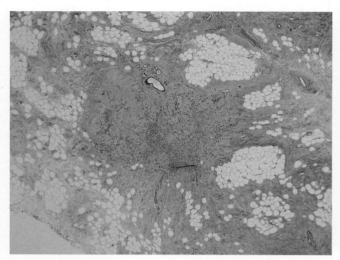

Figure 5.9.1 Sclerosing adenosis: Numerous small glandular structures are arranged in a lobulocentric configuration.

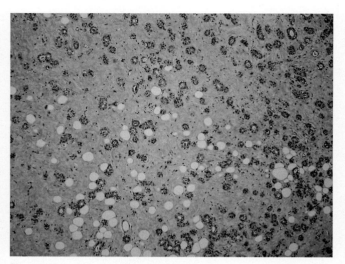

Figure 5.9.7 Microglandular adenosis characterized by small glandular structures arranged in a diffusely infiltrative pattern lacking lobulocentricity.

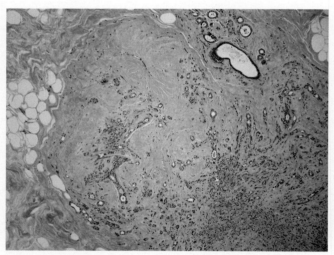

Figure 5.9.2 Dense, eosinophilic stroma deforms the acini in this example of sclerosing adenosis.

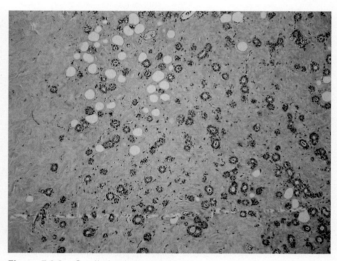

Figure 5.9.8 Small glands are present in unspecialized connective tissue and fat in microglandular adenosis.

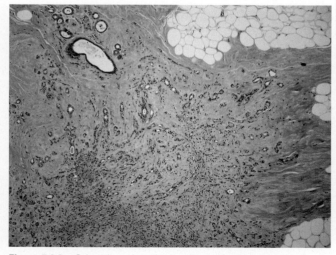

Figure 5.9.3 Sclerosing adenosis showing coalescence of several lobular units.

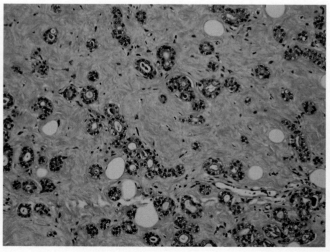

Figure 5.9.9 Glands are round and composed of a single cell layer in microglandular adenosis. The arrangement is not lobulocentric.

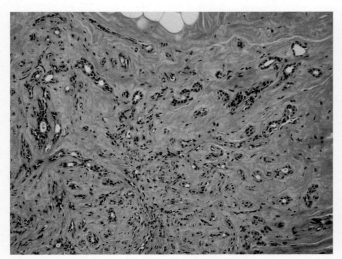

Figure 5.9.4   Glandular structures are associated with sclerotic intralobular stroma, resulting in compression of epithelium.

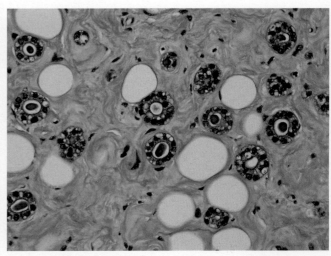

Figure 5.9.10   The glands of microglandular adenosis are round, composed of a single epithelial cell layer, and often contain eosinophilic secretory material. Myoepithelial cells are absent.

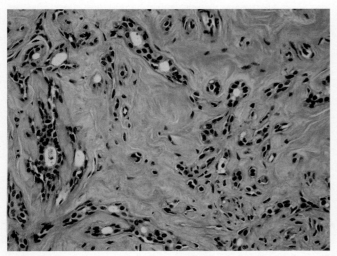

Figure 5.9.5   Small glandular structures maintain myoepithelial cells in this example of sclerosing adenosis.

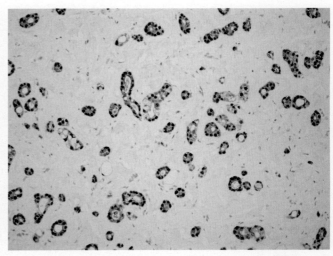

Figure 5.9.11   Immunohistochemical analysis shows strong, diffuse expression of S100 protein by microglandular adenosis.

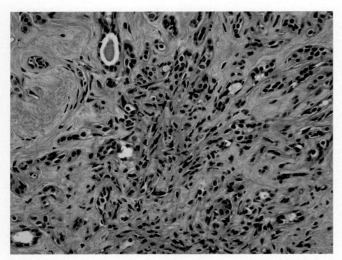

Figure 5.9.6   Sclerosis obliterates the lumens, and spindled myoepithelial cells are prominent in sclerosing adenosis.

SUGGESTED READINGS

Acs G, Simpson JF, Bleiweiss IJ, et al. Microglandular adenosis with transition into adenoid cystic carcinoma of the breast. *Am J Surg Pathol.* 2003;27:1052–1060.

Aroner SA, Collins LC, Connolly JL, et al. Radial scars and subsequent breast cancer risk: results from the Nurses' Health Studies. *Breast Cancer Res Treat.* 2013;139:277–285.

Brenner RJ, Jackman RJ, Parker SH, et al. Percutaneous core needle biopsy of radial scars of the breast: when is excision necessary?[see comment]. *Am J Roentgenol.* 2002;179:1179–1184.

Clement PB, Azzopardi JG. Microglandular adenosis of the breast—a lesion simulating tubular carcinoma. *Histopathology.* 1983;7:169–180.

Gobbi H, Simpson JF, Jensen RA, et al. Metaplastic spindle cell breast tumors arising within papillomas, complex sclerosing lesions, and nipple adenomas. *Mod Pathol.* 2003;16:893–901.

Hilson JB, Schnitt SJ, Collins LC. Phenotypic alterations in myoepithelial cells associated with benign sclerosing lesions of the breast. *Am J Surg Pathol.* 2010;34:896–900.

Jacobs TW, Byrne C, Colditz G, et al. Radial scars in benign breast-biopsy specimens and the risk of breast cancer. *N Engl J Med.* 1999;340:430–436.

James BA, Cranor ML, Rosen PP. Carcinoma of the breast arising in microglandular adenosis. *Am J Clin Pathol.* 1993;100:507–513.

Jensen RA, Page DL, Dupont WD, et al. Invasive breast cancer risk in women with sclerosing adenosis. *Cancer.* 1989;64:1977–1983.

Jones C, Tooze R, Lakhani SR. Malignant adenomyoepithelioma of the breast metastasizing to the liver. *Virchows Arch.* 2003;442:504–506.

Koenig C, Dadmanesh F, Bratthauer GL, et al. Carcinoma arising in microglandular adenosis: an immunohistochemical analysis of 20 intraepithelial and invasive neoplasms. *Int J Surg Pathol.* 2000;8:303–315.

Loose JH, Patchefsky AS, Hollander IJ, et al. Adenomyoepithelioma of the breast. A spectrum of biologic behavior. *Am J Surg Pathol.* 1992;16:868–876.

McLaren BK, Smith J, Schuyler PA, et al. Adenomyoepithelioma: clinical, histologic, and immunohistologic evaluation of a series of related lesions. *Am J Surg Pathol.* 2005;29:1294–1299.

Millis R. Microglandular adenosis of the breast. *Adv Anat Pathol.* 1995;2:10–19.

Page DL, Salhany KE, Jensen RA, et al. Subsequent breast carcinoma risk after biopsy with atypia in a breast papilloma. *Cancer.* 1996;78:258–266.

Rosen PP. Microglandular adenosis. A benign lesion simulating invasive mammary carcinoma. *Am J Surg Pathol.* 1983;7:137–144.

Sanders ME, Page DL, Simpson JF, et al. Interdependence of radial scar and proliferative disease with respect to invasive breast carcinoma risk in patients with benign breast biopsies. *Cancer.* 2006;106:1453–1461.

Simpson RH, Cope N, Skalova A, et al. Malignant adenomyoepithelioma of the breast with mixed osteogenic, spindle cell, and carcinomatous differentiation. *Am J Surg Pathol.* 1998;22:631–636.

Tavassoli FA. Myoepithelial lesions of the breast. Myoepitheliosis, adenomyoepithelioma, and myoepithelial carcinoma. *Am J Surg Pathol.* 1991;15:554–68.

Tavassoli FA, Norris HJ. Microglandular adenosis of the breast. A clinicopathologic study of 11 cases with ultrastructural observations. *Am J Surg Pathol.* 1983;7:731–737.

Wallis MG, Devakumar R, Hosie KB, et al. Complex sclerosing lesions (radial scars) of the breast can be palpable. *Clin Radiol.* 1993;48:319–320.

5 Papillary/Sclerosing

6

Invasive Carcinoma: Special Types and Important Considerations

	Pure Tubular Carcinoma	Radial Scar
Age	Any age, more often in postmenopausal women	Adult women, overlapping age with tubular carcinoma
Location	Anywhere in the breast	Anywhere in the breast
Presentation	Indistinguishable from no special type carcinomas; may be multifocal; frequently low stage (pT1) although may rarely may involve one or two low axillary lymph nodes	Usually mammographic abnormality, rarely palpable mass. May mimic invasive carcinoma clinically and radiographically
Imaging findings	Mammogram shows a spiculated mass, which may contain calcifications; up to one half may be incidental to calcifications associated with atypical hyperplasia or ductal carcinoma in situ (DCIS); hypoechoic mass with ill-defined margins and posterior acoustic shadowing on ultrasound	Mammography shows asymmetric density or architectural distortion, often with central translucence; hypoechoic mass or density, parenchymal distortion by ultrasound
Epidemiology	Approximately 2% of invasive breast cancers, more frequently detected (20%) by mammographic screening	Incidence unknown, although more common with high-quality mammography
Histology	1. Haphazard arrangement of small glandular structures *(Fig. 6.1.1)* 2. More than 90% of tumor consists of ovoid and "bent teardrop"-shaped tubules *(Fig. 6.1.2)* 3. Tubules composed of a single layer of cuboidal epithelial cells with low-grade nuclei and inconspicuous nucleoli *(Figs. 6.1.3 and 6.1.4)* 4. Apical snouts frequently present *(Fig. 6.1.4)* 5. In addition to tubules, a component of cribriform structures infiltrates basophilic, desmoplastic stroma with irregular extension into fat *(Fig. 6.1.5)* 6. Often seen in association with ADH, low-grade DCIS, ALH, or columnar cell lesions with atypia 7. By definition, tubular carcinoma has a low combined histologic grade	1. Radial arrangement of small glandular structures, emanating from central elastosis *(Fig. 6.1.6)* 2. Lobulocentric arrangement is maintained, and glandular structures do not infiltrate fat *(Fig. 6.1.7)* 3. Small glands are associated with dense periductal fibrosis, at least focally *(Fig. 6.1.8)* 4. Glands of radial scar maintain a myoepithelial and luminal cell layer *(Fig. 6.1.9)* 5. Myoepithelial cells may be detected by immunohistochemistry, although they may be sparse *(Fig. 6.1.10)*
Special studies	Strong expression of ER, usually expresses PR; uniformly lacks HER2 amplification. Myoepithelial cells not detected by immunohistochemistry.	Immunohistochemistry for myoepithelial cells may be helpful if present, but occasionally radial scars and other sclerosing lesions may lack myoepithelial cells; use of a battery of markers may be helpful

	Pure Tubular Carcinoma	**Radial Scar**
Genetics	16q loss (75%–85%), 1q gain (50%–60%); 16p gain, loss of 8p, 3p (*FHIT* locus) and 11q (*ATM* locus)	None
Treatment	Complete surgical excision is adequate therapy for most cases. Axillary dissection considered unnecessary even in presence of a positive sentinel node; in many cases radiation therapy unnecessary; chemotherapy is not indicated.	Often excised when diagnosed on core biopsy; however, if histology and mammography are concordant, and no risk lesions (i.e., atypical hyperplasia) are present, excision is not necessary
Clinical implication	Excellent prognosis even in the presence of a positive axillary lymph node(s); survival rates similar to the general population; risk of local recurrence extremely low after complete excision	Radial scars (and related complex sclerosing lesions) may mimic invasive carcinomas clinically and mammographically. Subsequent carcinoma risk is that attributed to any epithelial proliferation that may be present within the radial scar, i.e., usual hyperplasia or atypical hyperplasia. The radiology literature suggests that radial scars are a premalignant lesion; however, these studies have selection bias and lack of careful case definition.

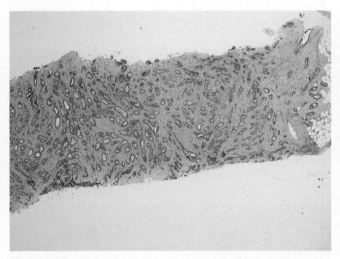

Figure 6.1.1 Tubular carcinoma, showing haphazard arrangement of small, angulated tubular structures.

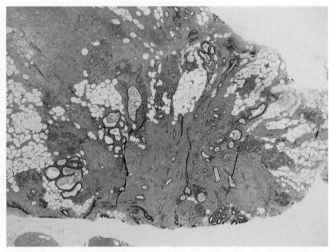

Figure 6.1.6 Glandular structures radiate from an elastotic center in a radial scar.

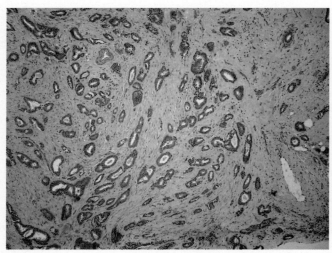

Figure 6.1.2 Tubular carcinoma characterized by open glands and occasional bent "tear drop" structures.

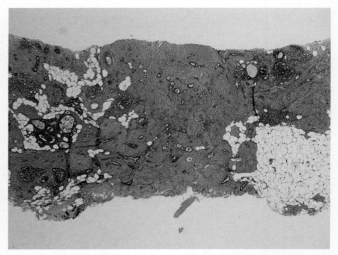

Figure 6.1.7 The glands of a radial scar maintain a lobulocentric configuration and do not extend into fat.

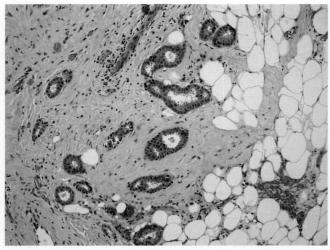

Figure 6.1.3 Small glands, some with occasional cribriform features, infiltrate fat in pure tubular carcinoma.

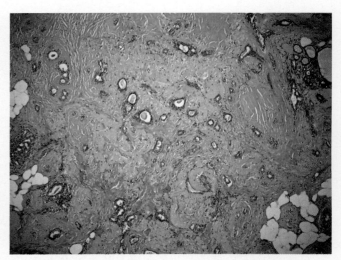

Figure 6.1.8 The glands of a radial scar lack the haphazard arrangement of tubular carcinoma; lobulocentricity is maintained, and elastosis is present around several of the ducts.

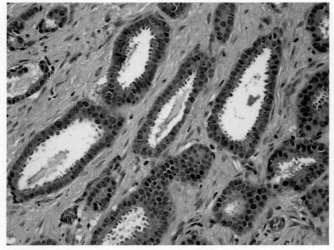

Figure 6.1.4 Glands of tubular carcinoma are lined by a single cell layer with minimal pleomorphism and apocrine snouts.

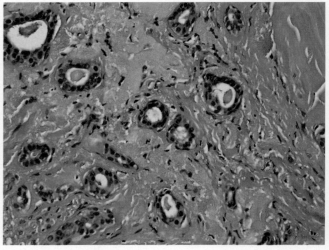

Figure 6.1.9 Two cell layers are present in radial scar.

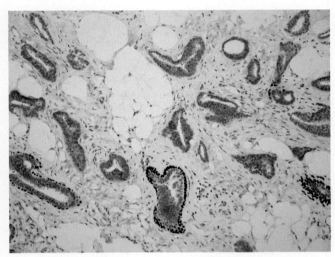

Figure 6.1.5 Immunohistochemistry using antibodies to p63 shows a lack of myoepithelial cells in tubular carcinoma; three normal ducts retain myoepithelial cells (lower center, right and left).

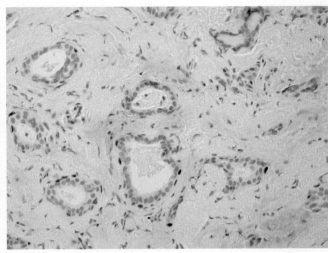

Figure 6.1.10 Immunohistochemistry using antibodies to p63 shows maintenance of myoepithelial cells in a patchy distribution.

	Invasive Cribriform Carcinoma	Cribriform Ductal Carcinoma In Situ
Age	Adult women, usually 6th decade	Most commonly middle-aged and older women, wide age range
Location	Anywhere in the breast	Anywhere in the breast
Presentation	Mammographic abnormality; rarely palpable mass	Mammographic abnormality, rarely clinically evident
Imaging findings	Spiculated mass, often with microcalcifications	Punctate or linear calcifications, rarely mass forming
Epidemiology	Less than 1.0% of invasive carcinomas; more commonly detected in screening programs; may be multifocal	20%–25% of screen detected breast cancers, 80%–85% detected in absence of clinical findings
Histology	1. Irregularly placed epithelial islands with cribriform spaces are present in a desmoplastic stroma *(Figs. 6.2.1 and 6.2.2)* with infiltration into fat *(Fig. 6.2.3)* 2. Tubular component may comprise up to 50% of tumor	1. Lobular units and true ducts contain a proliferation of uniform cells *(Fig. 6.2.4)* 2. Even cell placement results in rigid secondary spaces *(Fig. 6.2.5)* 3. Cribriform DCIS usually has a low or intermediate nuclear grade *(Fig. 6.2.6)*
Special studies	Strong expression of ER, usually expresses PR; uniformly lacks HER2 amplification. Myoepithelial cells not detected by immunohistochemistry.	None required; immunohistochemistry for myoepithelial markers may facilitate recognition of a noninvasive process when present
Genetics	16q loss (75%–85%), 1q gain (50%–60%); 16p gain; loss of 8p, 3p (FHIT locus) and 11q (ATM locus)	None to distinguish from low-grade invasive mammary carcinoma
Treatment	Complete surgical excision is adequate therapy for most cases. Axillary dissection considered unnecessary even in presence of a positive sentinel node; chemotherapy is not indicated.	Excision to negative margins ± radiation therapy; antiestrogen therapy may be indicated for some patients
Clinical implication	Excellent prognosis, even in the presence of a positive axillary lymph node(s); survival rates similar to that of pure tubular carcinoma, which is not different from the general population; risk of local recurrence extremely low after complete excision	Risk of local recurrence as DCIS or invasive carcinoma if excision incomplete

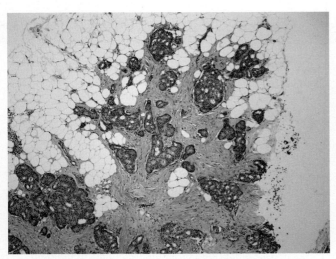

Figure 6.2.1   Broad tumor islands with cribriform architecture are irregularly arranged in invasive cribriform carcinoma.

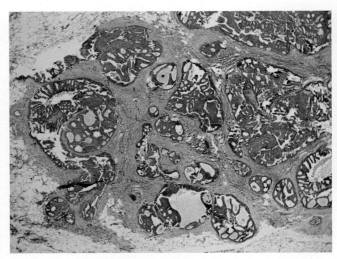

Figure 6.2.4   The original duct and lobular architecture are evident, despite the expansion and distortion by cribriform DCIS.

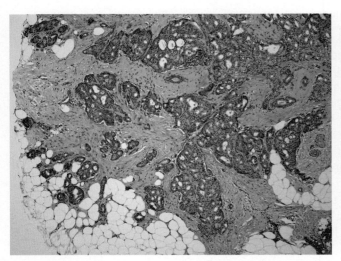

Figure 6.2.2   Cribriform glands have irregular shapes and do not conform to preexisting ductal lobular structures; note infiltration into fat (lower left).

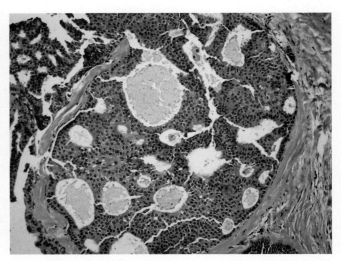

Figure 6.2.5   Uniform cells delineate crisp secondary spaces in low-grade cribriform DCIS.

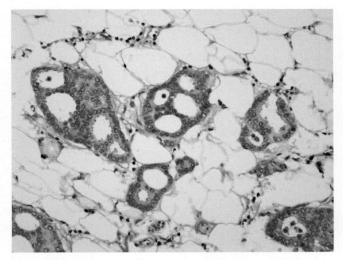

Figure 6.2.3   Invasive cribriform carcinoma with a focal tubular component. Despite superficial resemblance to cribriform DCIS, the cellular islands lack lobulocentricity and are irregularly distributed.

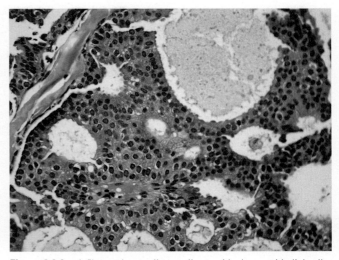

Figure 6.2.6   A fibrous duct wall as well as residual myoepithelial cells are evident in low-grade DCIS, cribriform pattern.

	Pure Mucinous Carcinoma	No Special Type Carcinoma with Mucin Production
Age	Middle-aged and older women; most patients older than 55 years	Middle-aged and older women; most patients older than 55 years
Presentation	Mammographic abnormality, less frequently presents as a palpable mass	Mammographic abnormality or palpable mass
Location	Anywhere in the breast	Anywhere in the breast
Imaging findings	Well-circumscribed lesion on mammography, frequently suggests a benign process; hypoechoic mass on ultrasound	Circumscribed or spiculated mass depending on amount of mucin present
Epidemiology	Approximately 2% of invasive breast cancers	Approximately 5% of invasive breast cancers
Histology	1. Small nests, trabeculae, or sheets of epithelial cells, which appear suspended in pools of extracellular mucin *(Fig. 6.3.1)* 2. Delicate fibrous septae containing capillaries are scattered throughout the mucin *(Fig. 6.3.2)* 3. Epithelial component must be of low nuclear grade and represent a minor component of the lesion; mitotic figures should not be evident *(Fig. 6.3.3)* 4. Must be at least 90% pure in pattern to diagnose pure mucinous carcinoma; any other minor component must be low grade	1. Nests, trabeculae, or sheets of intermediate- or high-grade carcinoma entirely or partially suspended in mucin *(Fig. 6.3.4)* 2. May show invasive micropapillary features *(Fig. 6.3.5)* 3. Mitotic figures may be frequent *(Fig. 6.3.6)*
Special studies	Strong expression of ER and PR; HER2 not amplified	Vary widely on intensity and extent of ER expression; subset shows HER2 amplification
Genetics	16q loss (75%–85%), 1q gain (50%–60%), similar to pure tubular carcinoma	Similar to other intermediate and high-grade, no special type invasive carcinomas
Treatment	Excision to negative margins ± radiation therapy, ± antiestrogen therapy; chemotherapy not indicated	Excision to negative margins + radiation therapy, chemotherapy frequently given; antiestrogen therapy if ER-positive
Clinical implication	10 year survival rates similar to age-matched controls without carcinoma (80%–100%)	Worse prognosis and higher rates of lymph node metastases compared with pure mucinous carcinoma

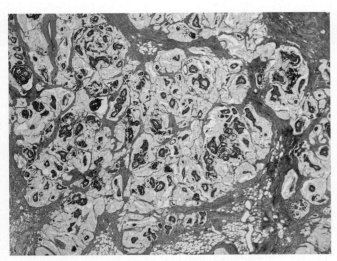

Figure 6.3.1   Small glandular structures appear suspended in extracellular mucin in pure mucinous carcinoma.

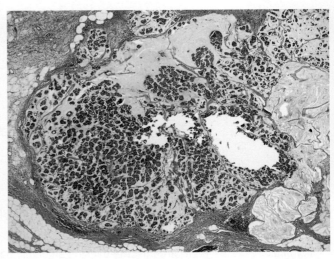

Figure 6.3.4   Invasive mammary carcinoma, no special type with extracellular mucin production: Although extracellular mucin is prominent, the degree of cellularity is too great to consider pure mucinous carcinoma.

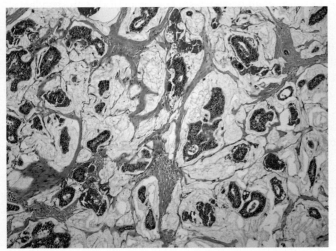

Figure 6.3.2   Delicate fibrovascular structures permeate pools of mucin in pure mucinous carcinoma.

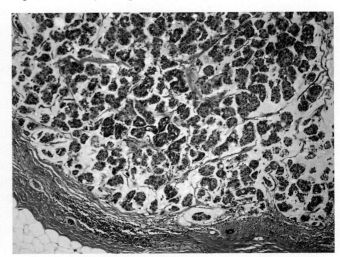

Figure 6.3.5   More than 50% of the tumor is composed of neoplastic epithelium, a feature that supports the diagnosis of invasive mammary carcinoma, no special type with extracellular mucin production, rather than pure mucinous carcinoma.

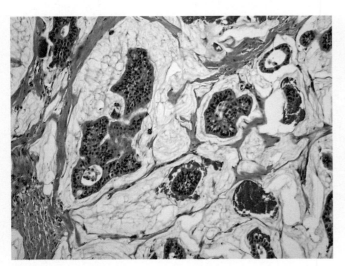

Figure 6.3.3   The paucicellular proliferation of pure mucinous carcinoma has a low nuclear grade without mitoses.

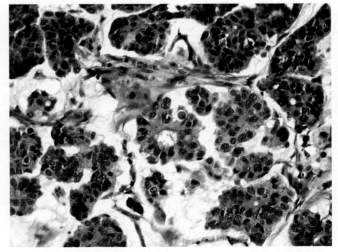

Figure 6.3.6   Grade 2 nuclei are not a feature of pure mucinous carcinoma. The amount of epithelium relative to the amount of mucin also supports the diagnosis of a no special type carcinoma with extracellular mucin production.

	Pure Mucinous Carcinoma	Mucocele-Like Lesion Associated with DCIS
Age	Middle-aged and older women, most patients older than 55 years	Any age, usually women in 5th and 6th decade
Location	Anywhere in the breast	Anywhere in the breast; if associated with intraductal papilloma, may be retroareolar
Presentation	Mammographic abnormality, less frequently presents as a palpable mass	Mammographic abnormality, rarely palpable mass or associated with bloody nipple discharge
Imaging findings	Well-circumscribed lesion on mammography, frequently suggesting a benign process; hypoechoic mass on ultrasound	Irregular density, may be associated with calcifications; ultrasound shows hypoechoic mass
Epidemiology	Approximately 2% of invasive breast cancers	Rare finding associated with DCIS with abundant mucin production
Histology	1. Small nests, trabeculae, or sheets of epithelial cells, which appear suspended in pools of extracellular mucin *(Fig. 6.4.1)*. By definition, mucinous carcinoma should be paucicellular 2. Delicate fibrous septae containing capillaries are present within mucin pools *(Fig. 6.4.2)* 3. Epithelial component must be of low nuclear grade and represent a minor component of the lesion; mitotic figures should not be evident *(Fig. 6.4.3)* 4. Must be at least 90% pure in pattern to diagnose pure mucinous carcinoma; any other minor component must be low grade	1. Traumatic or iatrogenic disruption of mucin-producing DCIS with extrusion of mucin and DCIS fragments into the surrounding stroma *(Fig. 6.4.4)* 2. Extracellular mucin follows contours of preexisting ducts *(Fig. 6.4.5)* 3. Some mucin pools contain a peripheral layer of epithelium *(Fig. 6.4.6)*, a remnant of a disrupted duct 4. Solid or cribriform architecture of DCIS maintained in extruded epithelial fragments containing uniform cells of low nuclear grade *(Figs. 6.4.5 and 6.4.6)*
Special studies	Uniformly expresses ER and PR; no amplification of HER2	None; myoepithelial cells maintained in epithelial fragments which remain associated with a basement membrane. ER expression routinely evaluated to assess the potential for response adjuvant endocrine therapy; multigene assay may predict which patients may be spared radiation.
Genetics	16q loss (75%–85%), 1q gain (50%–60%), essentially the same as pure tubular carcinoma	Loss of 16q, 17p
Treatment	Excision to negative margins ± radiation therapy, antiestrogen therapy; chemotherapy not indicated	Complete excision with negative margins, ± adjuvant radiation; sentinel lymph node biopsy not indicated
Clinical implication	10 y survival rates similar to age-matched controls without carcinoma	Development of invasive carcinoma in approximately 30% of cases if DCIS incompletely excised; with complete excision recurrence rate approximately 5%–8% without radiation

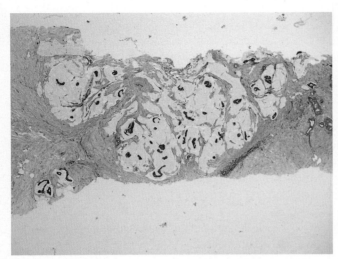

Figure 6.4.1   Pure mucinous carcinoma, with a characteristic bland, paucicellular epithelial component "floating" in extracellular mucin.

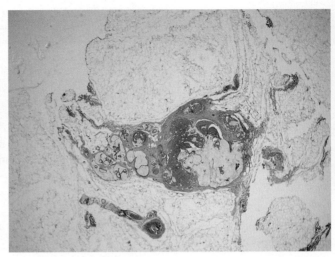

Figure 6.4.4   Low-grade DCIS with a mucocele-like lesion. An epithelial proliferation conforms to preexisting terminal ducts/lobular units and is associated with extracellular mucin.

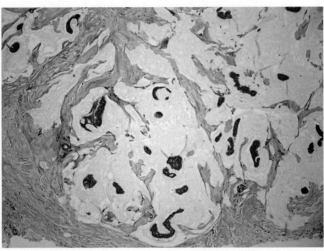

Figure 6.4.2   Thin fibrous strands containing capillaries traverse areas of mucin in pure mucinous carcinoma.

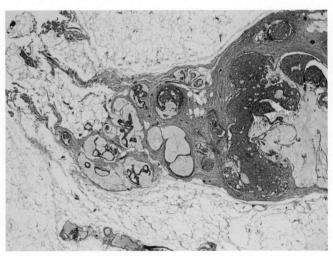

Figure 6.4.5   A solid, expansile nodule of low-grade DCIS has intermixed mucin. Epithelial disruption is also evident, although most collections of mucin are partially lined by ductal cells.

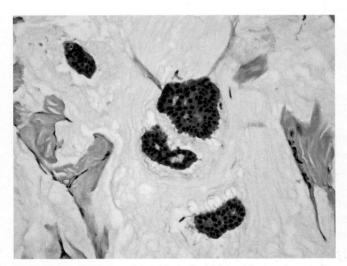

Figure 6.4.3   Grade 1 nuclei and lack of mitotic activity are characteristic of pure mucinous carcinoma.

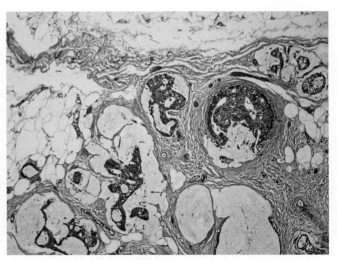

Figure 6.4.6   Expanded and disrupted ducts contain mucin, with residual ductal epithelium lining at least part of the mucin-filled spaces in this mucocele-like lesion associated with low-grade DCIS.

	Invasive Lobular Carcinoma	No Special Type Carcinoma with Lobular Features
Age	Women in 6th and 7th decade, slightly older than women with invasive mammary carcinoma of no special type	Women in 6th and 7th decade, slightly older than women with invasive mammary carcinoma of no special type
Location	Anywhere in the breast	Anywhere in the breast
Presentation	Ill-defined palpable mass or mammographic abnormality	Ill-defined palpable mass or palpable abnormality
Imaging findings	Spiculated mass or architectural distortion	Spiculated mass or architectural distortion
Epidemiology	5%–15% of invasive breast cancers	5%–15% of breast cancers
Histology	1. Single-file infiltration by neoplastic cells, comprises at least 90% of tumor *(Figs. 6.5.1 and 6.5.2)* 2. Residual normal ducts and lobular units may be present 3. Single-file growth of cells lacks cohesion *(Fig. 6.5.3)*. May encircle pre-existing structures in a "targetoid" pattern 4. Intracytoplasmic inclusions are frequent *(Fig. 6.5.4)* 5. Often nuclear grade 2, although mitotic activity is rare	1. Single-file growth pattern composes a portion of the carcinoma, but less than required for a diagnosis of pure invasive lobular carcinoma *(Fig. 6.5.5)*. Small cellular clusters and glands are also present. 2. Single-file growth may encircle preexisting structures, so-called "tagetoid" pattern, similar to pure invasive lobular carcinoma *(Fig. 6.5.6)* 3. Usually nuclear grade 2, and mitotic activity low *(Fig. 6.5.7)* 4. Small neoplastic glands and solid nests are intermixed with the neoplastic cells showing single-file growth *(Fig. 6.5.8)*
Special studies	None required for diagnosis; strongly ER-positive; invasive lobular carcinoma usually lacks expression of E-cadherin; p120 expression maintained	Usually ER-positive; loss of E-cadherin expression may be seen in lobular component
Genetics	Loss of 16q, contains locus for E-cadherin	16q loss, 1q gain
Treatment	Same as invasive carcinoma of no special type: neoadjuvant or adjuvant endocrine therapy, surgical excision to negative margins and adjuvant radiation therapy. Breast conservation not contraindicated. The single-file growth pattern may make obtaining clear surgical margins difficult, requiring mastectomy.	Adjuvant or neoadjuvant endocrine therapy, surgical excision to negative margins and adjuvant radiation; Adjuvant chemotherapy for higher grade lesions
Clinical implication	Stage and grade dictate prognosis. Prognosis intermediate between special types (tubular, cribriform, and mucinous) and carcinomas of no special type. Specific metastatic patterns often associated with ILC, including bone-only disease, spread to gastrointestinal tract, uterus, ovary, serosal surfaces and meninges as well as the occurrence of metastasis many years after treatment of the primary breast carcinoma.	Stage and grade dictate prognosis; lobular component may have similar pattern of spread as pure invasive lobular carcinoma

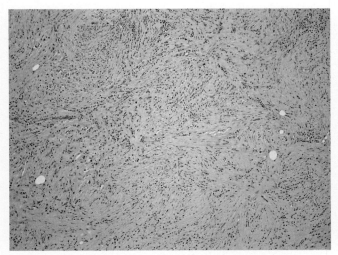

Figure 6.5.1   Invasive lobular carcinoma, characterized by diffuse single-file growth pattern.

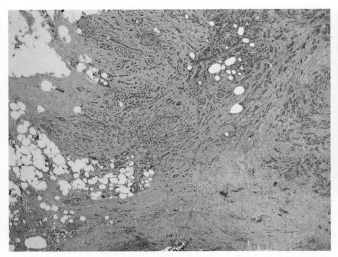

Figure 6.5.5   Although part of this invasive carcinoma has a single-file growth pattern, more than half of the tumor is composed of small nests and cords, denying a diagnosis of pure invasive lobular carcinoma.

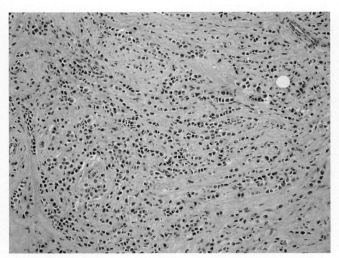

Figure 6.5.2   Invasive lobular carcinoma should be composed of at least 90% single-file growth pattern.

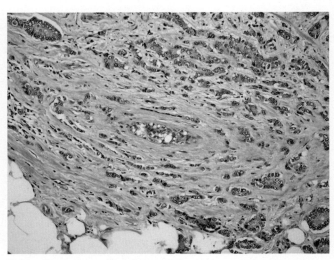

Figure 6.5.6   Targetoid growth pattern may be seen in invasive carcinoma, no special type with lobular features.

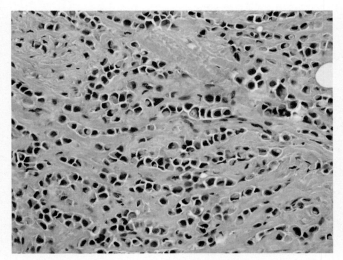

Figure 6.5.3   The morphologic correlate of lack of E-cadherin expression in invasive lobular carcinoma is its dyshesive growth.

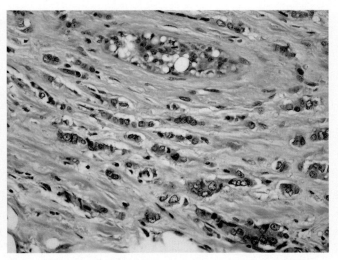

Figure 6.5.7   Grade 2 nuclei are present in strands and cords in this example of invasive carcinoma, no special type with lobular features.

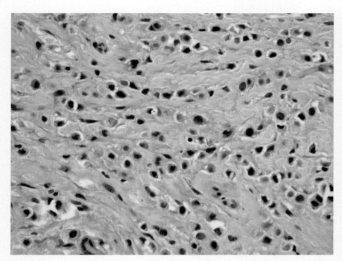

Figure 6.5.4   Nuclei are round and regular with minimal pleomorphism; intracytoplasmic inclusions are frequent in invasive lobular carcinoma.

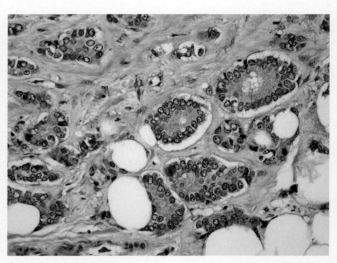

Figure 6.5.8   Solid nests and small glandular structures are admixed with tumor growing in a single file pattern, supporting the diagnosis of invasive carcinoma of no special type, with lobular features.

	No Special Type Carcinoma with Medullary Features	High-Grade, No Special Type Carcinoma with Associated Lymphocytic Infiltrate
Age	Any age, but often young women in 3rd and 4th decade	Any age, generally older than women with carcinomas showing medullary features
Location	Anywhere in the breast	Anywhere in the breast
Presentation	Often presents as a palpable mass or mammographic abnormality	Palpable mass or mammographic abnormality
Imaging findings	Nodular density; ultrasound shows a hypoechoic mass with smooth borders	Nodular density; ultrasound lacks smooth borders
Epidemiology	Less than 1% of breast cancers	30%–40% of high-grade, no special type carcinomas
Histology	1. Neoplastic epithelial proliferation associated with a smooth pushing border *(Fig. 6.6.1)* 2. Neoplastic epithelium must be arranged in a sheet-like (syncytial) growth pattern *(Fig. 6.6.2)* 3. Stroma between cellular syncytia contains a dense lymphoplasmacytic infiltrate *(Fig. 6.6.3)* 4. By definition, carcinomas with medullary features have a high combined histologic grade *(Fig. 6.6.4)*	1. Expansile growth pattern but lacks syncytial growth *(Fig. 6.6.5)* 2. Small nests of neoplastic cells infiltrate fat *(Fig. 6.6.6)* 3. Lymphocytic infiltrate present within tumor nests, rather than confined to stroma *(Fig. 6.6.7)* 4. High-grade nuclei and frequent mitoses are characteristic *(Fig. 6.6.8)*
Special studies	Negative for expression of ER and PR; HER2 not amplified	None to distinguish from medullary carcinoma; usually lacks expression of ER and PR; may be HER2 amplified
Genetics	Basal-like genomic profile; *TP53* mutations are most common alteration; *BRCA1* mutations frequent	*TP53* mutations most common alteration; ± *BRCA1* mutations
Treatment	Neoadjuvant chemotherapy followed by surgical excision is currently preferred therapy	Neoadjuvant chemotherapy followed by surgical excision
Clinical implication	Older literature supports good prognosis for node negative medullary carcinoma, although currently, concerns about reproducibility in applying criteria, triple-negative receptor status and frequent presentation in young women prompts administration of taxane chemotherapy	Prognosis based on stage, although high-grade, triple-negative carcinomas often have the poorest prognosis

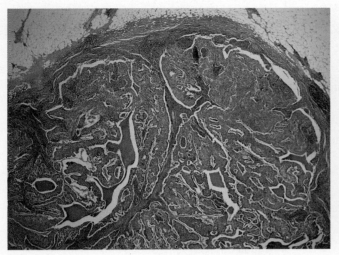

Figure 6.6.1   Carcinoma with medullary features, showing the characteristic smooth pushing border with adjacent fat.

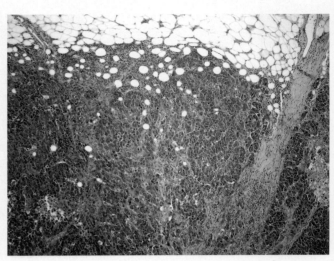

Figure 6.6.5   Invasive carcinoma, no special type, showing an overall rounded contour with adjacent fat, but neoplastic nests infiltrate fat in an irregular pattern.

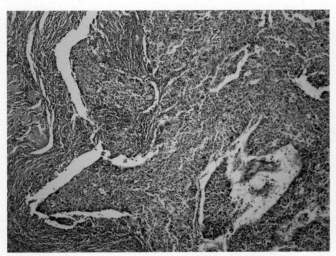

Figure 6.6.2   The diagnosis of carcinoma with medullary features requires a sheet-like (syncytial) growth pattern, with neoplastic epithelium separated by fibrous stroma containing lymphocytes and plasma cells.

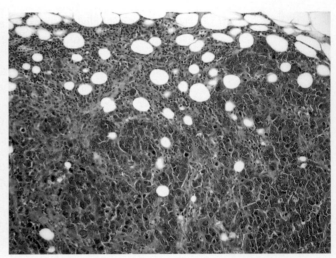

Figure 6.6.6   Invasive carcinoma, no special type showing small infiltrating glands, rather than syncytial growth.

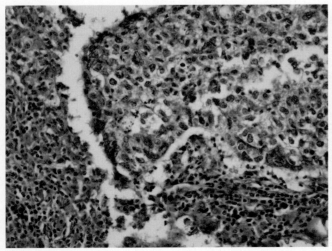

Figure 6.6.3   Lymphocytes and plasma cells are confined to the fibrous stroma and are not prominent within the epithelial sheets in carcinomas with medullary features.

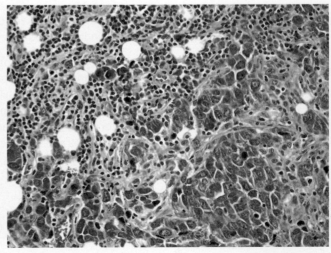

Figure 6.6.7   Invasive carcinoma, no special type, showing lymphocytes percolating within neoplastic nests, rather than confined to the adjacent fibrous stroma, as is required in carcinomas with medullary features.

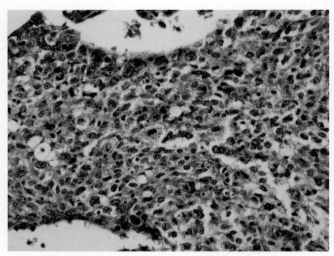

Figure 6.6.4 High nuclear grade and frequent mitotic activity are characteristic of carcinomas with medullary features.

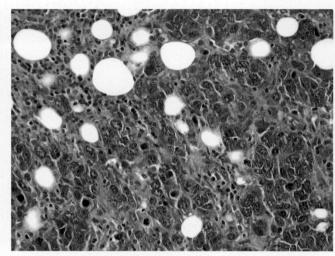

Figure 6.6.8 High-grade nuclei and frequent mitotic figures are present in this invasive carcinoma of no special type. Scattered lymphocytes are present, but the distribution and growth pattern are not defining for medullary carcinoma.

	Small Cell Carcinoma	No Special Type Carcinoma with Neuroendocrine Differentiation
Age	Adult women, mean age 65 years	Adult women, commonly 6th and 7th decade
Location	Anywhere in the breast	Anywhere in the breast
Presentation	Mammographic abnormality or palpable mass; up to 40% with metastatic disease at presentation	None to distinguish from no special type carcinomas without neuroendocrine differentiation; mammographic abnormality or palpable mass
Imaging findings	Spiculated mammographic mass	Indistinguishable from other no special type carcinomas
Epidemiology	Less than 1% of invasive breast cancers	Less than 1% of invasive breast carcinomas
Histology	1. Morphologically indistinguishable from small cell carcinoma of lung and other sites *(Fig. 6.7.1)* 2. Sheets and nests of diffusely infiltrating neoplastic associated with desmoplastic stroma *(Figs. 6.7.2 and 6.7.3)* 3. Hyperchromatic cells with scant cytoplasm *(Fig. 6.7.4)* 4. High mitotic activity, apoptotic bodies, focal necrosis, and crush artifact *(Fig. 6.7.4)* 5. DCIS component common 6. Associated lymphovascular invasion common	1. Cellular, solid nests and trabeculae of tumor cells in a fibrovascular stroma *(Figs. 6.7.5–6.7.8)* 2. Cells are spindled to plasmacytoid *(Figs. 6.7.6–6.7.8)* 3. Most are low or intermediate grade *(Fig. 6.7.8)*
Special studies	Half express chromogranin and synaptophysin; approximately 50% ER-positive	50% express chromogranin and 15% express synaptophysin; almost always ER-positive
Genetics	No distinguishing genetic features	No distinguishing genetic features
Treatment	High dose taxane-based chemotherapy and etoposide similar to that used for small cell carcinoma of the lung. Addition of radiation therapy does not improve survival.	Same as invasive carcinoma of no special type of same stage and grade; presence of neuroendocrine features is of no clinical significance
Clinical implication	Poorer prognosis than invasive mammary carcinoma of no special type of similar grade and stage	Prognosis depends on grade and stage

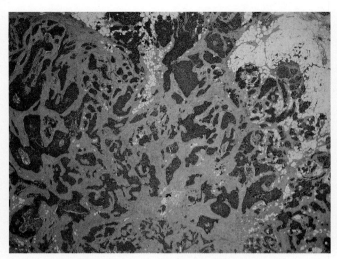

Figure 6.7.1 Small cell carcinoma: Infiltrating irregular islands of hyperchromatic cells are associated with desmoplastic stroma.

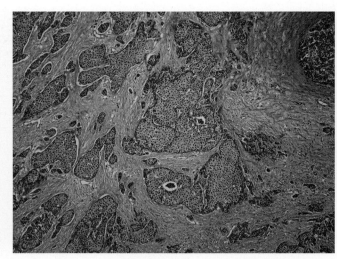

Figure 6.7.5 Sheets of neoplastic cells are associated with desmoplastic stroma in carcinoma of no special type with neuroendocrine features.

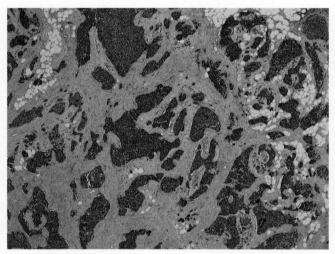

Figure 6.7.2 Small cell carcinoma: Infiltrating nests of neoplastic cells have a high nuclear to cytoplasmic ratio.

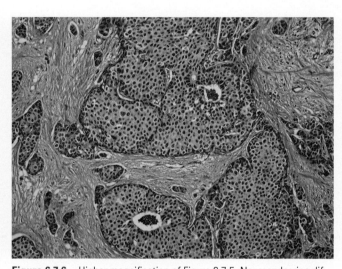

Figure 6.7.6 Higher magnification of Figure 6.7.5. Neuroendocrine differentiation is prominent, with microrosettes.

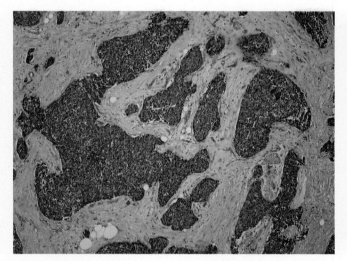

Figure 6.7.3 The undifferentiated cells of small cell carcinoma show focal crush artifact.

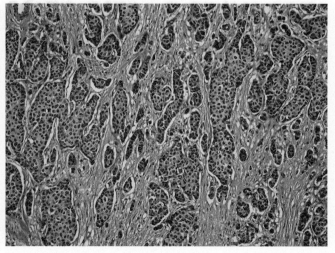

Figure 6.7.7 Trabecular growth pattern in no special type carcinoma with neuroendocrine features.

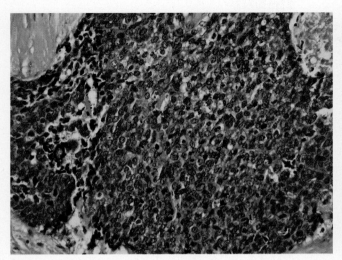

Figure 6.7.4 High nuclear to cytoplasmic ratio and crush artifact are characteristic of small cell carcinoma. Mitotic figures are frequent.

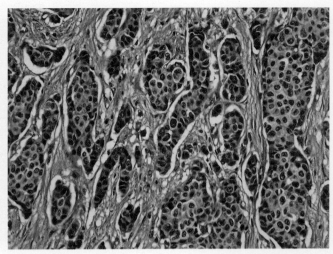

Figure 6.7.8 Cytoplasm is more abundant than in small cell carcinoma. Cytology is characteristic of carcinomas with neuroendocrine features.

	Adenoid Cystic Carcinoma	Cribriform Ductal Carcinoma In Situ
Age	65 years median age at diagnosis	Most commonly middle-aged and older women, wide age range
Location	50% subareolar	Mammographic abnormality, rarely clinically evident
Presentation	Firm subareolar mass, may be painful	Anywhere in the breast
Imaging findings	Irregular or lobulated mass mammographically, may have well defined borders; Hypoechoic solid or heterogeneous mass on ultrasound	Punctate or linear calcifications, rarely mass forming
Epidemiology	Rare, <0.1% of all breast carcinomas	20%–25% of screen detected breast cancers, 80%–85% detected in absence of clinical findings
Histology	1. Diffusely infiltrating rounded nests (Fig. 6.8.1) 2. Islands composed of a dual cell population with epithelial and myoepithelial cells forming small, sharply defined true and false lumens (Fig. 6.8.2) 3. True lumens are filled with brightly eosinophilic mucin, and false lumens contain basophilic basement membrane material (Figs. 6.8.2 and 6.8.3)	1. Lobular units and true ducts contain a proliferation of uniform cells (Fig. 6.8.4) 2. Even cell placement results in cribriform structures (Fig. 6.8.4) and microrosettes (Fig. 6.8.5) 3. Cribriform DCIS usually has a low or intermediate nuclear grade (Fig. 6.8.6)
Special studies	Epithelial component expresses cytokeratin, epithelial membrane antigen, and c-kit (CD117); myoepithelial component expresses p63 and actin. No expression of ER or PR; HER2 not amplified. Alcian blue-PAS stains the contents of the "true" lumens pink (neutral mucin) and basement membrane material in "false lumens" blue (acidic mucin).	None required; immunohistochemistry for myoepithelial markers may facilitate recognition of a noninvasive process
Genetics	Recurrent translocation t(6;9)(q22–23;p23–24) with resultant *MYB-NFIB* fusion transcript present in >90% of cases; somatic mutations of *PIK3CA* and *PTEN* reported	None to distinguish from low-grade invasive mammary carcinoma
Treatment	Complete excision curative in most cases, radiotherapy and chemotherapy not indicated	Excision to negative margins ± radiation therapy; ± antiestrogen therapy
Clinical implication	Despite "triple-negative" status and frequent mitotic activity, adenoid cystic carcinoma is associated with an excellent prognosis in the breast	Risk of local recurrence as DCIS or invasive carcinoma if excision incomplete

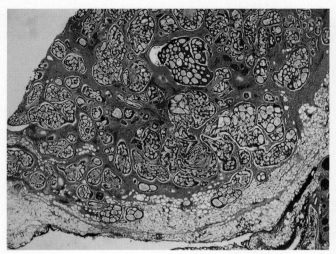

Figure 6.8.1   Adenoid cystic carcinoma, composed of diffusely infiltrating rounded nests of cells that maintain cribriform architecture.

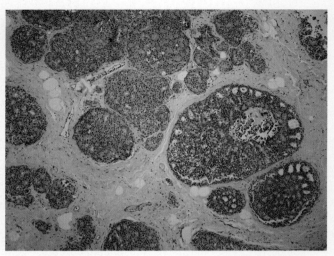

Figure 6.8.4   Terminal duct lobular units are expanded by a proliferation of cells forming cribriform spaces in low-grade DCIS. A lobulocentric configuration is maintained.

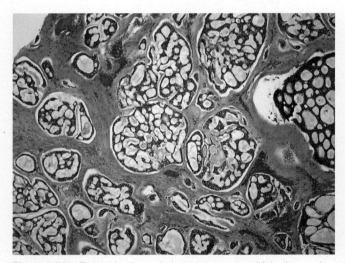

Figure 6.8.2   The dual cell population creates true and false lumens in adenoid cystic carcinoma.

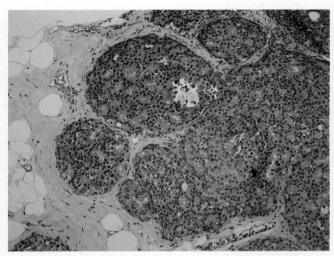

Figure 6.8.5   In addition to cribriform architecture, microrosettes are frequent in DCIS.

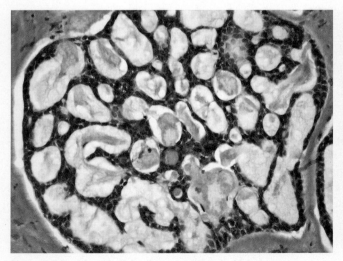

Figure 6.8.3   Moepithelial cells are associated with basement membrane material within false lumens, while luminal epithelium surrounds true lumens containing mucin.

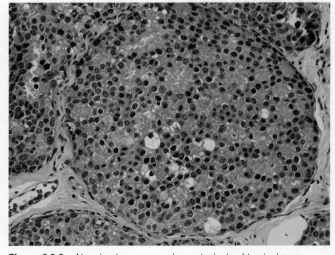

Figure 6.8.6   Neoplastic nests consist exclusively of luminal type epithelium, bounding cribriform spaces and creating microrosettes in cribriform DCIS.

	Adenoid Cystic Carcinoma	Collagenous Spherulosis
Age	65 years median age at diagnosis	Adult women
Location	50% subareolar	Anywhere in the breast
Presentation	Firm subareolar mass, may be painful	Incidental finding
Imaging findings	Irregular or lobulated mass mammographically, may have well defined borders; hypoechoic solid or heterogeneous mass on ultrasound	None
Epidemiology	Rare, <0.1% of all breast carcinomas	Unknown
Histology	1. Diffusely infiltrating rounded nests *(Fig. 6.9.1)* 2. Islands composed of a dual cell population with epithelial and myoepithelial cells forming small, sharply defined true and false lumens *(Fig. 6.9.2)* 3. True lumens are filled with brightly eosinophilic mucin, and false lumens contain basophilic basement membrane material *(Figs. 6.9.2 and 6.9.3)*	1. Terminal ducts and lobular units contain spherules composed of basement membrane material that mimics cribriform spaces *(Fig. 6.9.4)* 2. True and false lumens are present, and epithelium appears "stretched" around spherules of basement membrane *(Figs. 6.9.5 and 6.9.6)* 3. Luminal epithelial cells border true lumens *(Fig. 6.9.6)* 4. True lumens contain neutral mucin (blue staining on alcian blue/PAS stain), false lumens contain acidic mucin (pink staining on alcian blue/PAS stain), reflective of basement membrane material
Special studies	Epithelial component expresses cytokeratin, epithelial membrane antigen and c-kit (CD117); myoepithelial component expresses p63 and actin. No expression of ER or PR; HER2 not amplified. Alcian blue-PAS stains the contents of the "true" lumens pink (neutral mucin) and basement membrane material in "false lumens" blue (acidic mucin).	Alcian blue/PAS or immunohistochemistry to detect basement membrane material
Genetics	Recurrent translocation t(6;9)(q22–23;p23–24) with resultant *MYB-NFIB* fusion transcript present in >90% of cases; somatic mutation of *PIK3CA* and *PTEN* reported	Unknown
Treatment	Complete excision curative in most cases, radiotherapy and chemotherapy not indicated	None
Clinical implication	Despite "triple-negative" status and frequent mitotic activity, adenoid cystic carcinoma in the breast is associated with an excellent prognosis	None

143

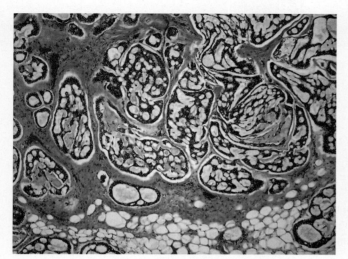

Figure 6.9.1   Adenoid cystic carcinoma showing diffusely infiltrating islands.

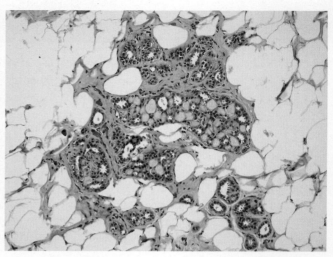

Figure 6.9.4   A lobular unit contains an epithelial proliferation with prominent cribriform architecture in this example of collagenous spherulosis.

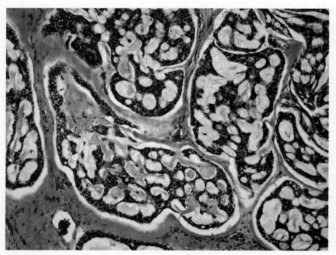

Figure 6.9.2   Dual cell population defines the true and false lumens of adenoid cystic carcinoma.

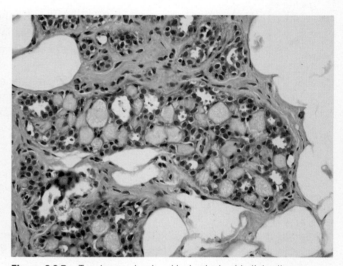

Figure 6.9.5   True lumens bordered by luminal epithelial cells are associated with false lumens composed of basement membrane material in collagenous spherulosis.

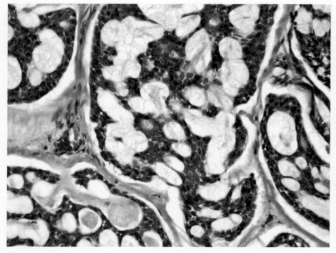

Figure 6.9.3   False lumens contain pink basement membrane material while true lumens contain wispy secretions in this example of adenoid cystic carcinoma.

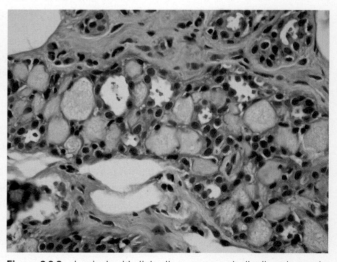

Figure 6.9.6   Luminal epithelial cells are not evenly distributed around all lumens, but appear "stretched" around basement membrane material in collagenous spherulosis.

	Secretory Carcinoma	No Special Type Carcinoma with Secretory Features
Age	Originally described in children and adolescents (juvenile carcinoma), although there is a wide age range (3–87 y); median age 25 y	Adult women, most commonly 6th and 7th decades, wide age range
Location	Anywhere in the breast	Anywhere in the breast
Presentation	Well-circumscribed mass near areola	Mammographic abnormality or palpable mass
Imaging findings	Circumscribed mass mammographically; on ultrasound, hypoechoic mass with circumscribed or infiltrative edges	Spiculated mass on mammogram; mass with irregular margins, taller than wide on ultrasound, similar to invasive carcinomas of no special type
Epidemiology	Less than 0.5% of invasive breast cancers, occurs in both sexes	Rare, incidence unknown
Histology	1. Infiltrative tumor islands with a microcystic appearance separated by prominant bands of densely sclerotic collagen *(Figs. 6.10.1 and 6.10.2)* 2. Numerous intercellular lumina contain extracellular eosinophilic secretions *(Fig. 6.10.3)* 3. Tumor islands composed of cells with low-grade nuclei *(Fig. 6.10.3)*	1. Diffusely infiltrating glands containing bubbly cytoplasm and luminal secretions *(Figs. 6.10.4)* 2. Infiltrating glands are not separated by eosinophilic collagenous stroma *(Fig. 6.10.4 and 6.10.5)* 3. Tumor is composed of cells with intermediate- or high-grade nuclei with mitotic figures *(Fig. 6.10.6)*
Special studies	Negative for expression of ER and PR, and HER2 is not amplified; secretory material both within tumor cells and within the intercellular lumina stains with PAS (diastase resistent) and Alcian blue	Commonly expresses ER
Genetics	t(12;15)(p12;q26.1) identified in adult and pediatric tumors. The resulting *ETV6-NTRK3* fusion gene encodes a chimeric tyrosine kinase with potent transforming activity in fibroblasts.	Absence of t(12;15)(p12;q26.1); none to distinguish from other no special type carcinomas
Treatment	Complete excision; adjuvant chemotherapy and radiation not indicated in young patients	Treated as other invasive carcinomas of no special type, based on stage, grade, hormone receptor status and HER2 expression
Clinical implication	In young patients, both male and female, less than 20 y old, the prognosis is excellent, despite "triple-negative" immunophenotype, even with axillary nodal involvement. In older patients, the clinical course may be more aggressive but sometimes protracted with distant recurrences occurring as late as 20 y after the primary diagnosis.	Prognosis depends on grade, stage, hormone receptor status, and HER2 expression

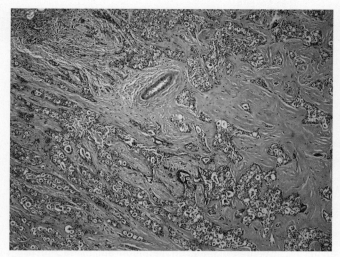

Figure 6.10.1 Secretory carcinoma: Epithelial nests with a microcystic appearance are diffusely infiltrative and separated by prominant bands of densely eosinophilic stroma.

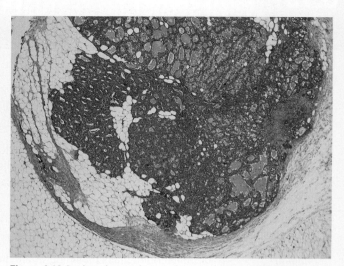

Figure 6.10.4 Invasive carcinoma of no special type, showing secretory features, including cytoplasmic inclusions and amphophilic luminal secretions.

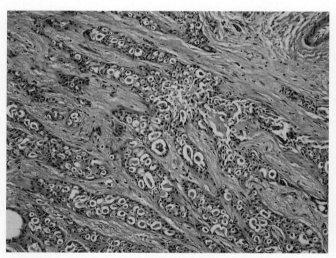

Figure 6.10.2 Tumor nests in secretory carcinoma are composed of cells with intracytoplasmic inclusions as well as extracellular secretions.

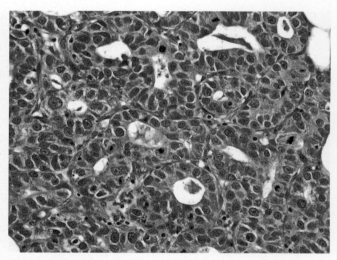

Figure 6.10.5 Carcinoma of no special type with secretory features. Diffuse infiltration by neoplastic glands without associated eosinophilic stroma.

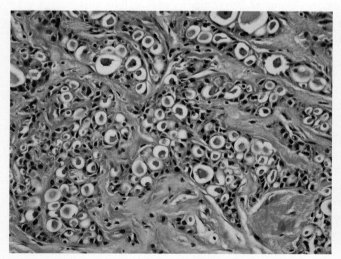

Figure 6.10.3 Low-grade nuclei and prominent eosinophilic secretory material are characteristic of secretory carcinoma.

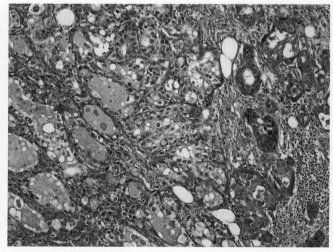

Figure 6.10.6 Nuclei are of intermediate grade, and mitotic activity is evident in this example of carcinoma of no special type, showing secretory features.

	Low-Grade Adenosquamous Carcinoma Associated with Sclerosed Papilloma	Papilloma with Squamous Morules Entrapped in Previous Biopsy Site
Age	Adult women	Adult women
Location	Anywhere in breast, but often subareolar	Anywhere in the breast, often subareolar
Presentation	Palpable mass or mammographic abnormality	Palpable mass, mammographic abnormality, or bloody nipple discharge
Imaging findings	Nodular density or spiculated mass on mammography; solid mass with irregular margins on ultrasound	Nodular density on mammography, solid and cystic mass on ultrasound
Epidemiology	Unknown	Unknown
Histology	1. Remnant of sclerotic intraductal papilloma usually present centrally (Figs. 6.11.1 and 6.11.2) 2. Infiltrating glandular structures emanate from central sclerotic papilloma (Fig. 6.11.2) 3. Small clusters of squamoid epithelial cells are mixed with bland spindle cells (Fig. 6.11.3) 4. Spindle cells, squamoid clusters, and glandular structures infiltrate beyond the confines of the papilloma into fat (Figs. 6.11.4 and 6.11.5)	1. Intraductal papilloma with adjacent fibroblastic reaction (Fig. 6.11.6) 2. Fibrovascular cores associated with bland epithelium (Fig. 6.11.7) 3. Dense fibroblastic proliferation, adjacent to duct lining (Fig. 6.11.8) 4. Degenerating squamous morules entrapped in dense fibrous scar (Fig. 6.11.9) 5. Squamous morules are associated with chronic inflammation, hemosiderin, and dense scar (Fig. 6.11.10)
Special studies	Immunohistochemistry using antibodies to high molecular weight cytokeratins and p63 highlight neoplastic squamoid clusters and spindled cells, the latter component is often inconspicuous using hematoxylin and eosin; negative for expression of ER and PR; HER2 not amplified	None required
Genetics	Gains 7p and 8q; loss 1p, 8p, 9p; subset with high level gains of *EGFR* (7p11.2)	None
Treatment	Complete excision; adjuvant radiation and chemotherapy are not indicated	Excision of intraductal papilloma is curative
Clinical implication	Capacity for local recurrence only	Documentation of previous biopsy helpful to avoid over diagnosing squamous morules

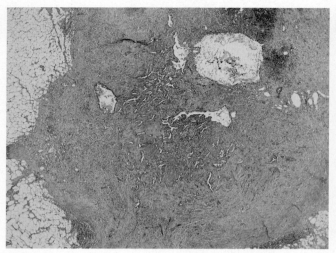

Figure 6.11.1   Low-grade adenosquamous carcinoma, with characteristic nodule of spindle cells surrounding a central remnant of sclerotic intraductal papilloma.

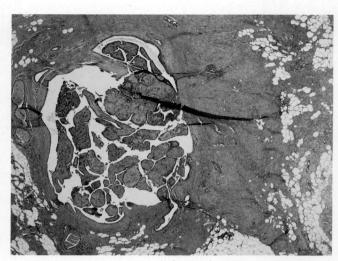

Figure 6.11.6   This sclerotic intraductal papilloma is surrounded by dense fibrous tissue.

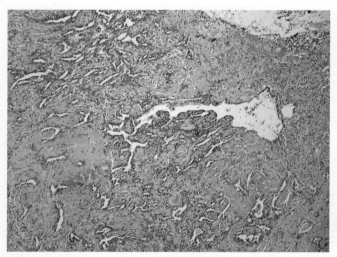

Figure 6.11.2   Irregular glandular structures emanate from a sclerotic papilloma in low-grade adenosquamous carcinoma.

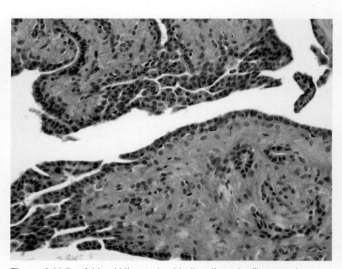

Figure 6.11.7   A bland bilayered epithelium lines the fibrovascular cores in this intraductal papilloma.

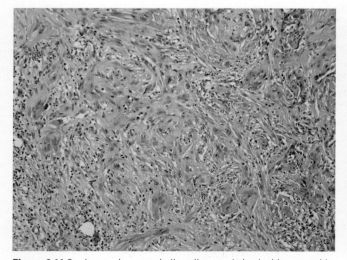

Figure 6.11.3   Inconspicuous spindle cells are admixed with squamoid clusters in low-grade adenosquamous carcinoma.

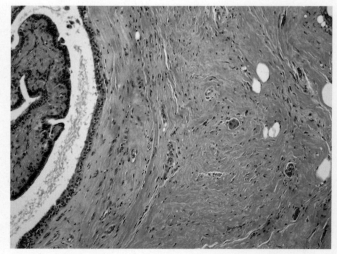

Figure 6.11.8   Surrounding the papilloma is dense scar, containing chronic inflammation.

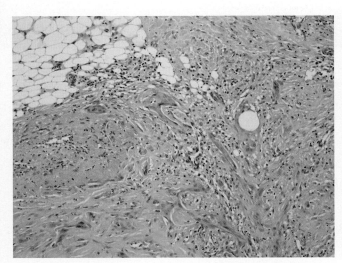

Figure 6.11.4   The neoplastic spindled and squamoid cells infiltrate fat in adenosquamous carcinoma.

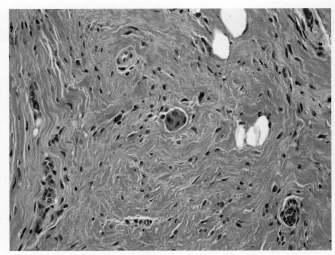

Figure 6.11.9   Degenerating squamous morules are entrapped in the dense scar of this previously biopsied intraductal papilloma.

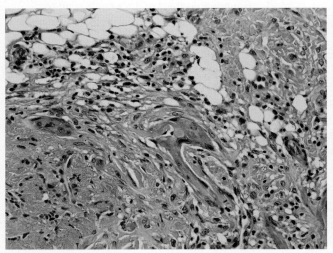

Figure 6.11.5   Irregular squamoid clusters are associated with chronic inflammation and spindle cells; the latter are often quite prominent using high molecular weight cytokeratin immunohistochemistry.

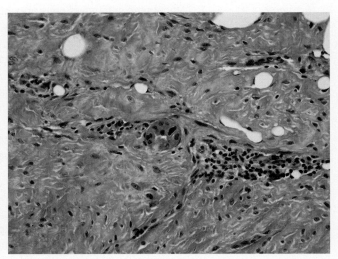

Figure 6.11.10   Pyknotic nuclei indicate degenerative change in this example of a previously biopsied intraductal papilloma with entrapped epithelium. Myoepithelial markers are not useful in this setting because of disruption and entrapment of epithelium.

	Squamous Cell Carcinoma	Squamous Metaplasia
Age	Any age, often in older women	Women of any age
Location	Any location, often subareolar	Anywhere in the breast
Presentation	Palpable mass, mammographic abnormality	Often associated with previous needle biopsy procedure
Imaging findings	Mammographic nodular density; cystic mass with irregular margins on ultrasound	Nodular density, rarely palpable
Epidemiology	Unknown	Sequelae of previous biopsy procedure or trauma
Histology	1. Neoplastic squamous cells present as sheets or as lining cystic cavity *(Fig. 6.12.1)* 2. DCIS, solid type with squamous cytology often present *(Fig. 6.12.2)* 3. Nests of malignant squamous cells have intermediate- or high-grade nuclei *(Fig. 6.12.3)* 4. Cytoplasm of malignant cells is densely eosinophilic, characteristic of squamous differentiation *(Fig. 6.12.4)*	1. Rounded contour of duct containing remnant of a sclerosed intraductal papilloma is often present *(Fig. 6.12.5)* 2. Squamous proliferation can be exuberant *(Fig. 6.12.6)* 3. Lobulated islands and nests of squamous cells confined by the encysting fibrous duct wall *(Fig. 6.12.6)* 4. Squamous cells show mild spongiosis *(Figs. 6.12.7 and 6.12.8)* 5. Nuclei demonstrate round to ovoid nuclei with a prominent nucleolus and mild reactive atypia *(Fig. 6.12.8)*
Special studies	Squamous cell carcinoma strongly expresses high molecular weight cytokeratins and p63; lacks expression of ER and PR; HER2 not amplified	None to distinguish from squamous cell carcinoma
Genetics	*TP53* and *PIK3CA* mutations, *PTEN* mutation or loss	No recurrent abnormalities reported
Treatment	Complete excision, adjuvant chemotherapy ineffective	None
Clinical implication	Poor prognosis with 65% progression-free survival at 5 y. Most failures from distant metastases.	None

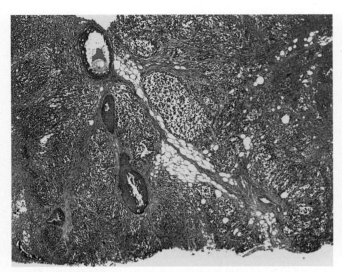

Figure 6.12.1 Squamous cell carcinoma: Sheets of infiltrating eosinophilic cells are associated with a squamous cell carcinoma in situ component.

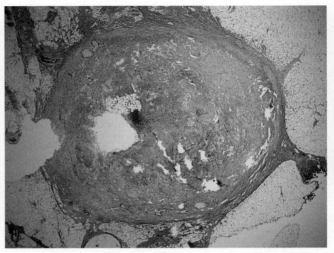

Figure 6.12.5 A nodule surrounded by dense collagen representing a remnant of an intraductal papilloma is a frequent setting for reactive squamous metaplasia.

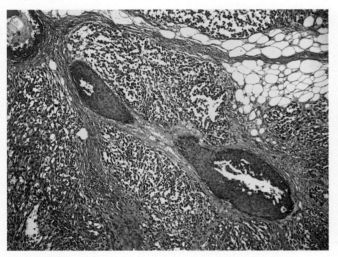

Figure 6.12.2 Squamous cell carcinoma composed of sheets of dyshesive cells.

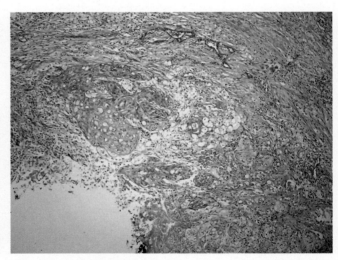

Figure 6.12.6 This exuberant reactive squamous proliferation is confined by the encysting fibrous wall of the pre-exising intraductal papilloma.

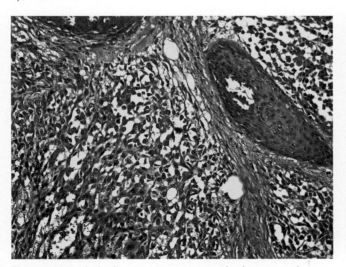

Figure 6.12.3 An in situ squamous component is often present in examples of squamous cell carcinoma.

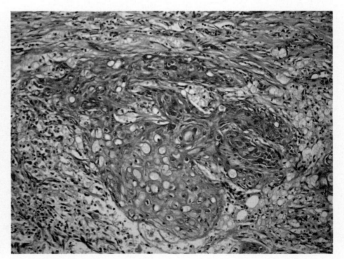

Figure 6.12.7 Sheets of reactive squamous cells show abundant cytoplasm and spongiosis.

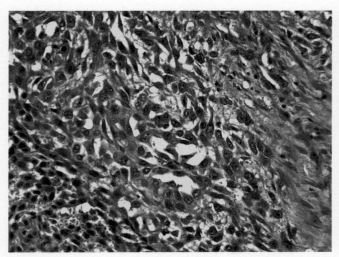

Figure 6.12.4   Densely eosinophilic cytoplasm characteristic of squamous cells, with a dyshesive growth pattern characterizes squamous cell carcinoma.

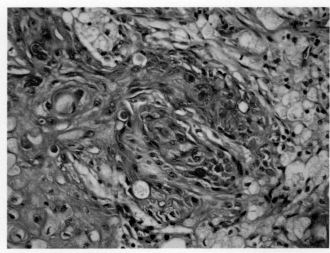

Figure 6.12.8   Reactive squamous metaplasia resembles the proliferating squamous epithelium in pseudoepitheliomatous hyperplasia in other sites.

6.13

DCIS INVOLVING CLUSTERED PAPILLOMAS WITH ASSOCIATED INVASION VS. DCIS INVOLVING CLUSTERED PAPILLOMAS WITH PSEUDOINVASION

	DCIS Involving Clustered Papillomas with Associated Invasion	DCIS Involving Clustered Papillomas with Pseudoinvasion
Age	Adult women, most commonly in 7th and 8th decades	Adult women
Location	Anywhere in the breast	Anywhere in the breast, often subareolar
Presentation	Mammographic abnormality, palpable mass, bloody nipple discharge	Mammographic abnormality, palpable mass, bloody nipple discharge; history of prior biopsy
Imaging findings	Architectural distortion ± an associated mass or masses	Architectural distortion ± an associated mass or masses
Epidemiology	Less than 1% of breast cancers	Less than 1% of breast cancers
Histology	1. The invasive epithelial elements infiltrate beyond the duct wall containing the papilloma *(Figs. 6.13.1–6.13.4)* 2. Invasive glands extend into unspecialized connective tissue *(Figs. 6.13.2 and 6.13.3)* 3. The irregular invasive edge which focally permeates fat contrasts with the smooth contour of the duct with DCIS *(Figs. 6.13.3 and 6.13.4)* 4. Invasive carcinoma component is usually of low or intermediate combined histologic grade *(Fig. 6.13.3)*	1. DCIS most commonly cribriform pattern, involves multiple ducts and papillomas *(Figs. 6.13.5–6.13.8)* 2. Neoplastic epithelial elements confined to papillomas, true ducts, and lobular units. 3. Detached fragments of DCIS resulting from prior biopsy are entrapped in granulation tissue and scar, and associated with hemosiderin *(Figs. 6.13.6–6.13.8)* 4. DCIS fragments have pyknotic nuclei, crush artifact, and degenerative changes *(Figs. 6.13.7 and 6.13.8)*
Special studies	Immunohistochemistry for myoepithelial markers frequently not useful as papilloma and invasive carcinoma can show loss of expression	None; myoepithelial markers may be helpful if positive; however, myoepithelial cells may be lost if displaced fragments are separated from the basement membrane
Genetics	Loss of heterozygosity at 16q and 1q reported; *PIK3CA* mutations	None to distinguish from invasive carcinoma
Treatment	Excision to negative margins ± radiation; antiestrogen therapy if invasive component is ER positive; sentinel lymph node biopsy indicated	Excision to negative margins ± radiation therapy; antiestrogen therapy may be indicated for ER-positive lesions
Clinical implication	T-stage based on size of invasive component only	Risk of local recurrence as DCIS or invasive carcinoma if excision incomplete; classified as pTis

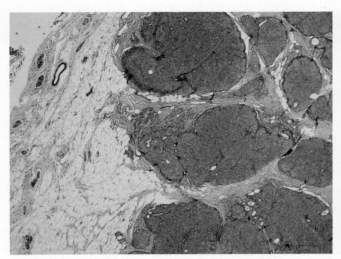

Figure 6.13.1   A solid, uniform proliferation of epithelial cells is present in this example of low-grade DCIS involving clustered intraductal papillomas.

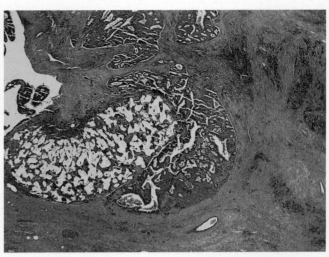

Figure 6.13.5   Intraductal papilloma with gel foam, characteristic of previous biopsy site.

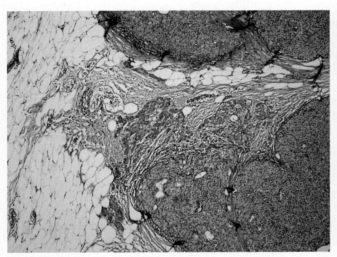

Figure 6.13.2   Invasive carcinoma arising in the setting of clustered papillomas involved by DCIS. Small irregular nests of cells infiltrate fat, beyond the confines of the papilloma.

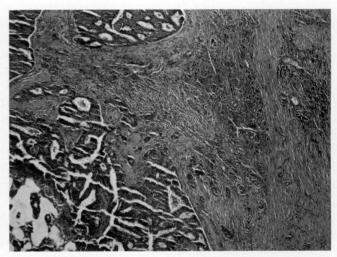

Figure 6.13.6   Fibroblastic reaction with blood, contains disrupted epithelium secondary to previous biopsy procedure. Several of the disrupted epithelial clusters remain associated with fragments of fibrovascular cores.

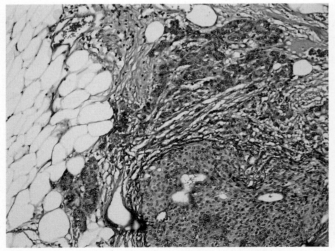

Figure 6.13.3   Small irregular clusters of carcinoma infiltrate stroma and are not associated with granulation tissue or hemosiderin.

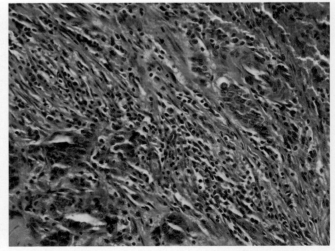

Figure 6.13.7   Epithelium entrapped in granulation tissue, following needle core biopsy procedure.

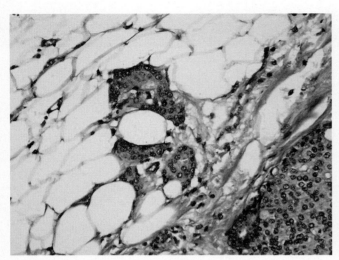

Figure 6.13.4   Fat infiltration by carcinoma arising in the setting of DCIS involving intraductal papillomas.

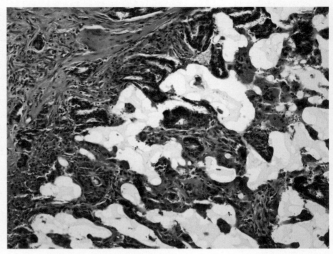

Figure 6.13.8   Disrupted epithelium associated with granulation tissue and blood. Immunohistochemical studies to detect myoepithelial cells in this setting are not useful, because disrupted epithelium often lacks myoepithelial cells.

	Carcinoma with Solid Pattern	Solid-Pattern Ductal Carcinoma In Situ
Age	Adult women, most commonly in 7th and 8th decades	Middle-age women, most commonly 40–60 years
Location	Anywhere in the breast	Anywhere in the breast
Presentation	Mammographic mass, palpable mass	Mammographic abnormality, palpable mass
Imaging findings	Spiculated mass, architectural distortion	Architectural distortion $\pm$ mass lesion; calcifications
Epidemiology	Rare pattern of invasive carcinoma, true incidence unknown	Uncommon pattern of DCIS in pure form, <10% of DCIS
Histology	1. Haphazard arrangement of solid tumor nests *(Figs. 6.14.1–6.14.3)* 2. Nonlobulocentric architectural pattern *(Figs. 6.14.1 and 6.14.2)* 3. Associated desmoplastic tumor stroma *(Fig. 6.14.3)* 4. Focal fatty infiltration and retraction *(Fig. 6.14.3)* 5. Invasion of lobular unit by malignant glands *(Fig. 6.14.4)*	1. True ducts and terminal duct lobular units are filled and distorted by a uniform population of epithelial cells *(Figs. 6.14.5–6.14.8)* 2. Within the membrane-bound spaces, cell placement is even and individual cell membranes are evident *(Figs. 6.14.6–6.14.8)* 3. Most involved spaces lack intercellular lumina, but subtle microrosettes may be seen *(Fig. 6.14.8, upper left)* 4. Usually low to intermediate nuclear grade
Special studies	Immunohistochemistry for myoepithelial markers may be helpful	Immunohistochemistry for myoepithelial markers may be helpful if present
Genetics	None unique to solid pattern	None specific to solid pattern
Treatment	Treated according to grade, stage, and hormone receptor status; excision to negative margins; radiation therapy; antiestrogens for ER-positive lesions	Excision to negative margins $\pm$ radiation therapy; antiestrogen therapy may be indicated for ER-positive lesions
Clinical implication	Prognosis based on grade, stage, hormone receptors and HER2 status	Risk of local recurrence as DCIS or invasive carcinoma if excision incomplete

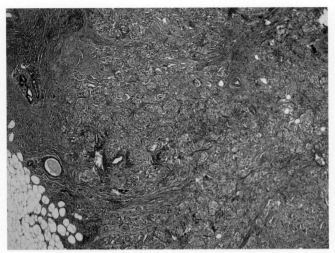

Figure 6.14.1 Invasive carcinoma of no special type with solid growth pattern: Small rounded nests of cells diffusely infiltrate stroma.

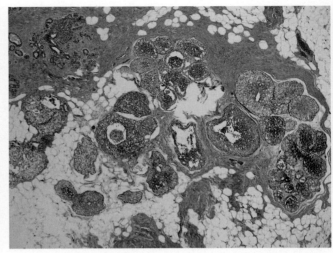

Figure 6.14.5 Solid-pattern DCIS characterized by an epithelial proliferation involving terminal ducts, lobular units, and true ducts.

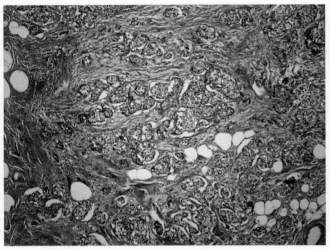

Figure 6.14.2 Invasive carcinoma lacks a lobulocentric configuration.

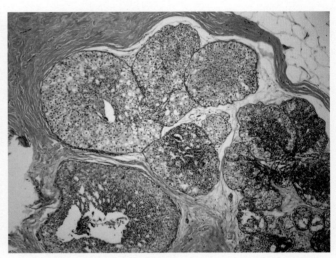

Figure 6.14.6 Solid-pattern DCIS expanding the involved lobular unit.

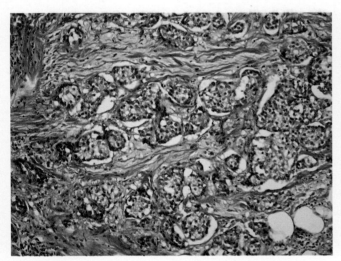

Figure 6.14.3 Low-grade carcinoma of no special type, showing infiltration into fat.

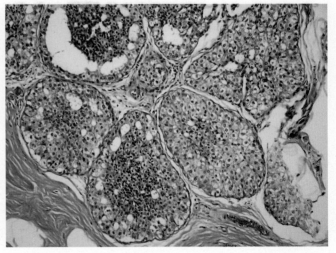

Figure 6.14.7 A lobulocentric arrangement is maintained in this example of DCIS involving lobular units.

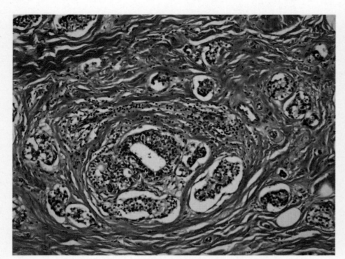

Figure 6.14.4   Small nests of infiltrating carcinoma encircle a preexisting terminal duct.

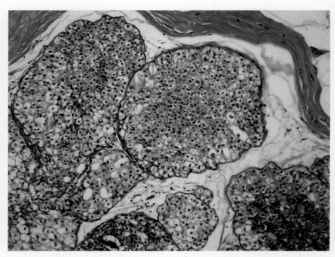

Figure 6.14.8   This lobular unit is greatly expanded by solid-pattern DCIS.

	Lymphovascular Invasion	Ductal Carcinoma In Situ
Age	Middle-aged women, most commonly 40–60 y	Most commonly middle-aged and older women, wide age range
Location	Anywhere in the breast	Anywhere in the breast
Presentation	Mammographic abnormality; often predicts axillary lymph node involvement; skin changes of inflammatory breast cancer if extensive involvement of dermal lymphatics	Mammographic abnormality, less commonly mass or bloody nipple discharge
Imaging findings	None specific to lymphovascular invasion	Punctate or linear calcifications, rarely mass forming
Epidemiology	Occurs in 10% of invasive carcinomas	20%–25% of screen detected breast cancers, 80%–85% detected in absence of clinical findings
Histology	1. Serpentine fragments of tumor are present in clear spaces but do not conform to the contours of the spaces *(Figs. 6.15.1–6.15.3)* 2. The dilated lymphatics containing tumor can often be recognized by their clustering with small veins and arterioles *(Fig. 6.15.2, right of center)* 3. Endothelial cells can frequently be recognized lining the irregular spaces *(Fig. 6.15.3)* 4. Most commonly associated with high-grade invasive carcinoma, but may be present in association with any grade	1. Lobular units and true ducts contain a proliferation of uniform cells without any evidence of retraction from the basement membrane *(Figs. 6.15.4–6.15.6)* 2. Normal ductal-lobular architecture is maintained *(Fig. 6.15.4)* 3. Ducts and acini filled with DCIS have smooth contours, and tumor cells are closely opposed to the basement membranes of the spaces *(Fig. 6.15.6)* 4. Foci of DCIS with solid patterns are those most likely to mimic LVI
Special studies	None routinely needed; immunohistochemistry may delineate vascular endothelium or lymphatic channels, e.g., CD31 or D2-40, lining the clear spaces	None required; immunohistochemistry for myoepithelial markers may facilitate recognition of a noninvasive process
Genetics	No known alterations correlate specifically with lymphovascular invasion	None to distinguish from low-grade invasive mammary carcinoma
Treatment	Treated according to grade, stage, and receptor status; excision to negative margins; radiation therapy; ± antiestrogen and/or chemotherapy	Excision to negative margins ± radiation therapy; antiestrogen therapy may be indicated for ER-positive lesions
Clinical implication	More frequently associated with metastasis to axillary lymph nodes and subsequent distant metastasis than cases without this feature. Predicts a worse prognosis than similar cases without peritumoral lymphovascular invasion.	Risk of local recurrence as DCIS or invasive carcinoma if excision incomplete

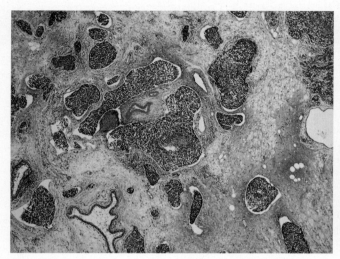

Figure 6.15.1   Extensive lymphovascular space involvement by carcinoma; this solid epithelial proliferation lacks a lobulocentric arrangement.

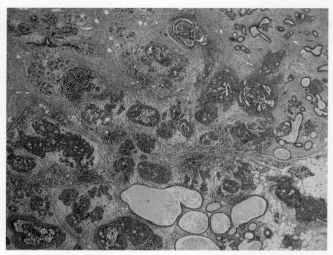

Figure 6.15.4   Solid-pattern DCIS, diffusely involving terminal ducts, lobular units, and true ducts.

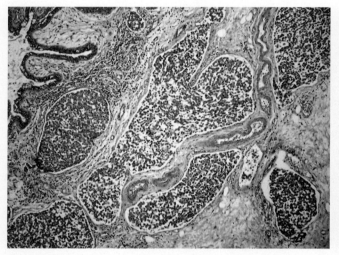

Figure 6.15.2   Solid tumor nests adjacent to arterioles and venules is the characteristic location for lymphovascular space involvement by carcinoma.

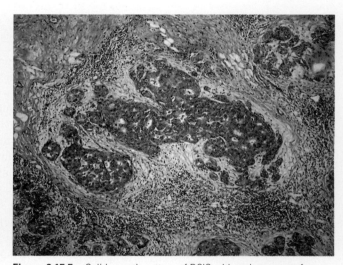

Figure 6.15.5   Solid growth pattern of DCIS with maintenance of a lobulocentric configuration.

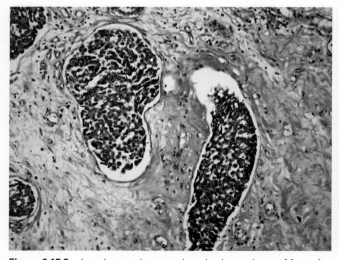

Figure 6.15.3   Lymphovascular space invasion by carcinoma. Many of the lymphovascular spaces are lined by endothelial cells.

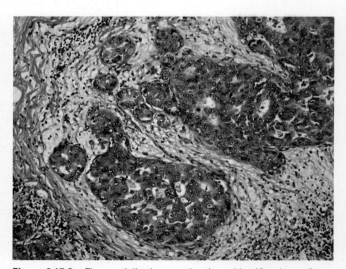

Figure 6.15.6   The specialized connective tissue identifies the confines of this lobular unit involved by DCIS.

	Invasive Micropapillary Carcinoma	Invasive Carcinoma with Retraction Artifact
Age	Same as women with ER-positive invasive mammary carcinoma of no special type	Adult women
Location	Anywhere in the breast	Anywhere in the breast
Presentation	Palpable mass or mammographic lesion	Palpable mass or mammographic lesion
Imaging findings	Dense mass with irregular or spiculated margins; hypoechoic, irregular, or microlobulated mass on ultrasound	Dense mass with irregular or spiculated margins. Hypoechoic, irregular, or microlobulated mass on ultrasound
Epidemiology	Rare in pure form representing 1%–2% of invasive mammary carcinomas; invasive micropapillary features in 8% of all invasive mammary carcinomas	Same as invasive carcinoma without this feature; 75%–80% of breast cancers diagnosed based on mammographic screening; 95% of palpable breast cancers
Histology	1. Invasive carcinoma composed of small clusters of cancer cells surrounded by clear spaces *(Fig. 6.16.1)* 2. Tumor cell nests display reverse polarity often referred to as the "inside-out" pattern in which the apical surface of the tumor cells face the stroma and lacks fibrovascular cores *(Fig. 6.16.2)* 3. Tumors cells are cuboidal *(Fig. 6.16.3)* 4. Most are intermediate or high combined histologic grade *(Fig. 6.16.3)* 5. Approximately 60% ER-positive, 30% HER2 overexpressing/amplified	1. Nests of invasive tumor often in desmoplastic stroma *(Fig. 6.16.5)* 2. Neoplastic cells may be partially attached to the basement membrane, with adjacent empty space formed by retraction artifact *(Figs. 6.16.6 and 6.16.7)* 3. Empty spaces lack an endothelial lining *(Fig. 6.16.8)*
Special studies	Epithelial membrane antigen (EMA) stains the apical surface of the tumor cells, highlighting the reversed polarity of the tumor cells; stain not required for diagnosis routinely *(Fig. 6.16.4)*	None routinely used; immunohistochemstry shows absence of expression of markers of vascular endothelium or lymphatic channels, e.g., CD31 or D2-40
Genetics	Recurrent gains of 8q, 17q, and 20q and deletions of 6q and 13q; recurrent amplifications of *MYC* (33%), *CCND1* (8%), and *FGFR1* (17%)	None reported related to retraction
Treatment	Treated according to grade, stage, and receptor status; excision to negative margins	Treated according to grade, stage, and receptor status; excision to negative margins
Clinical implication	Lymphovascular invasion and lymph node metastases more common than invasive carcinomas of no special type without invasive micropapillary features. Prognosis similar to patients with stage-matched invasive carcinoma of no special type.	None; does not convey worse prognosis

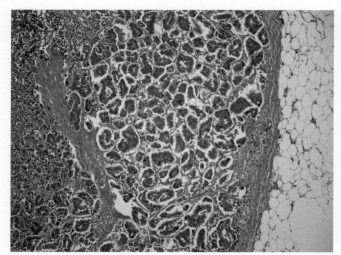

Figure 6.16.1   Invasive micropapillary carcinoma: The stroma is diffusely infiltrated by small clusters of cells associated with cleared spaces.

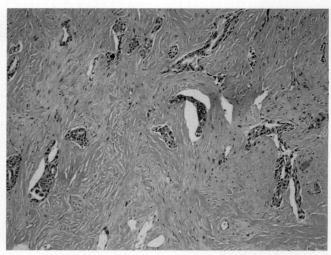

Figure 6.16.5   Invasive carcinoma of no special type, present in dense desmoplastic stroma showing retraction artifact around tumor nests.

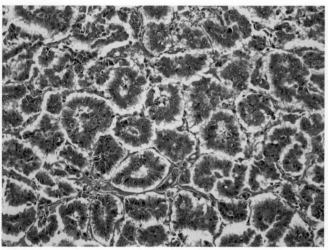

Figure 6.16.2   Invasive micropapillary carcinoma with characteristic "inside-out" morphology of tumor nests.

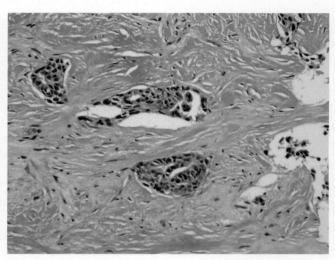

Figure 6.16.6   Retraction artifact associated with invasive carcinoma of no special type: Carcinoma is present in spaces that lack endothelial cells and do not have the orderly arrangement of the spaces that characterize invasive micropapillary carcinoma.

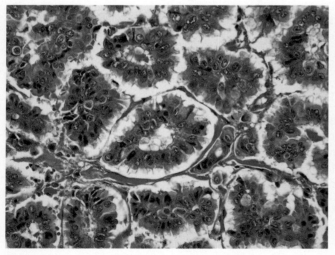

Figure 6.16.3   Invasive micropapillary carcinoma, showing luminal-type epithelial changes at the periphery of the tumor nests. Cleared spaces lack markers of lymphatic spaces, but are an essential component of this unusual invasive carcinoma.

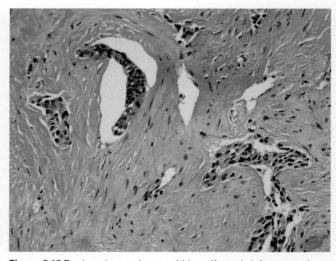

Figure 6.16.7   Invasive carcinoma within artifactual clefts present in desmoplastic stroma.

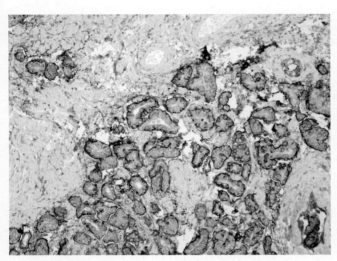

Figure 6.16.4 "Inside-out" arrangement of invasive micropapillary carcinoma highlighting the distribution of epithelial membrane antigen at the periphery of the nests.

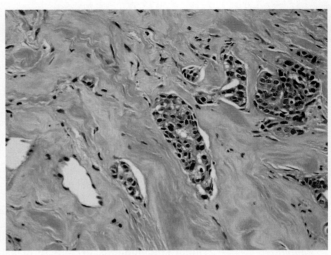

Figure 6.16.8 Invasive carcinoma associated with spaces secondary to retraction artifact, lacking an endothelial lining; note adjacent endothelial-lined lymphatic spaces.

	Microinvasive Carcinoma Associated with Ductal Carcinoma In Situ	Ductal Carcinoma In Situ in Lobular Units
Age	Same as DCIS without invasion	Not significantly different from women with DCIS accompanied by microinvasion
Location	Anywhere in the breast	Anywhere in the breast
Presentation	Usually mammographic abnormality, rarely bloody nipple discharge or mass	Mammographic abnormality, rarely bloody nipple discharge or mass
Imaging findings	Linear calcifications, architectural distortion, possibly mass lesion	Architectural distortion and calcifications, evidence of a mass lesion far less common than in cases with microinvasion
Epidemiology	Uncommon, frequently microinvasion is overdiagnosed	20%–25% of screen detected breast cancers, 80%–85% detected in absence of clinical findings
Histology	1. Associated DCIS may be any grade, most commonly seen in association with high-grade DCIS accompanied by prominent periductal fibrosis and chronic inflammatory infiltrate *(Fig. 6.17.1)* 2. Focus (foci) of infiltrative glands or solid nests of tumor in unspecialized connective tissue measuring no more than 1.0 mm *(Fig. 6.17.2)* 3. Irregular infiltration beyond the confines of the terminal duct lobular unit *(Figs. 6.17.3 and 6.17.4)*	1. DCIS involves or completely replaces acini of a lobular unit, recognized by a smooth, rounded interface with the surrounding stroma and maintenance of lobulocentricity at low power *(Figs. 6.17.5–6.17.8)* 2. Myoepithelial cells intact
Special studies	Immunohistochemistry for myoepithelial cells (p63, calponin, etc.) shows loss of expression, although only useful if DCIS maintains expression. It should be recalled that noninvasive sclerosing lesions may lose myoepithelial cell expression.	Immunohistochemistry for p63 highlights myoepithelial cells and emphasizes maintenance of lobulocentricity
Genetics	None to distinguish from DCIS	None to distinguish from microinvasion
Treatment	Treat as DCIS with consideration of sentinel lymph node biopsy, although risk of spread to axillary lymph nodes is low (9.4%)	Excision to negative margins ± radiation therapy; ± anti-estrogen therapy
Clinical implication	Prognosis excellent and not significantly different from women with pure DCIS of the same size and grade	Risk of local recurrence as DCIS or invasive carcinoma if excision incomplete

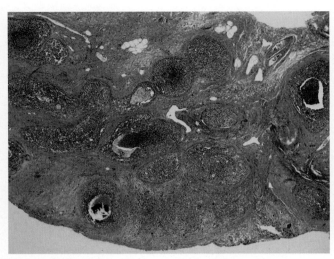

Figure 6.17.1   Solid growth pattern of DCIS, showing central necrosis and calcification.

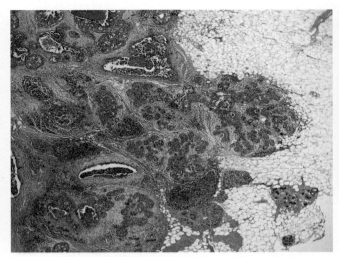

Figure 6.17.5   Solid growth pattern of DCIS: Terminal ducts, lobular units, and true ducts are expanded by a neoplastic proliferation.

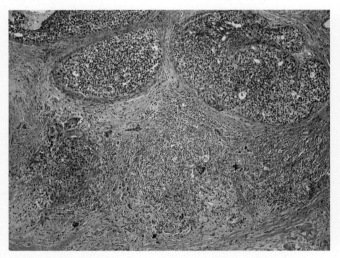

Figure 6.17.2   Microinvasive carcinoma, adjacent to solid pattern DCIS. Irregular cell clusters are associated with desmoplasia and chronic inflammation.

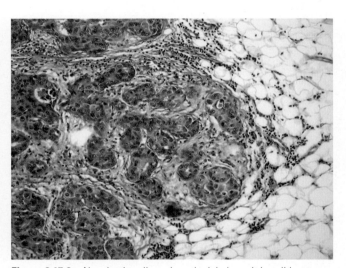

Figure 6.17.6   Neoplastic cells replace the lobular unit in solid-pattern DCIS.

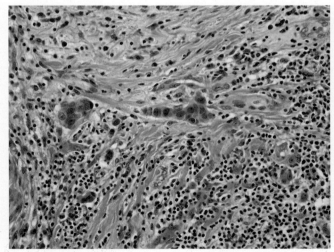

Figure 6.17.3   Microinvasive carcinoma: Infiltrating cell clusters are present beyond the specialized connective tissue of a lobular unit and lack a lobulocentric configuration.

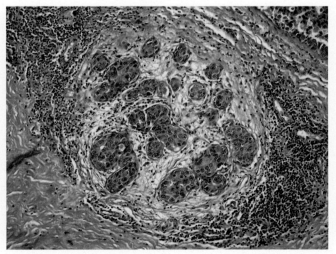

Figure 6.17.7   The neoplastic cells of the DCIS are confined to preexisting acini, without infiltration of specialized connective tissue or adjacent interlobular stroma.

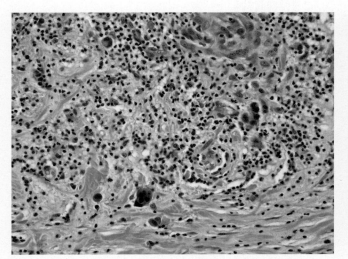

Figure 6.17.4   Microinvasive carcinoma: Small cellular clusters and individual cells infiltrate the stroma in an area measuring less than 1.0 mm.

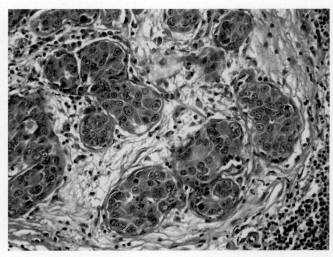

Figure 6.17.8   A lobular unit involved by DCIS: Although typically unnecessary for diagnosis, myoepithelial markers would be expected to be maintained in this setting.

	Invasive Carcinoma	DCIS Involving Sclerosing Adenosis
Age	Average age 60 y (usual range 45–75 y)	Any age, adult women
Location	Anywhere in the breast	Anywhere in the breast
Presentation	Mammographic or palpable mass	Mammographic abnormality, occasionally palpable mass
Imaging findings	Spiculated mass on mammography	Architectural distortion, microcalcifications, and/or mass lesion
Epidemiology	75%–80% of breast cancers diagnosed based on mammographic screening; 95% of palpable breast cancers; associated with family history, previous diagnosis of DCIS or atypical hyperplasia	20%–25% of breast cancers diagnosed based on mammographic screening; 2%–3% of palpable breast cancers
Histology	1. Haphazardly arranged glands, single cells, nests, islands or cords of tumor; lobulocentric architecture lost *(Figs. 6.18.1–6.18.4)*	1. DCIS involves a sclerosing process with maintenance of lobulocentricity at low power *(Fig. 6.18.5)* 2. Malignant cells partially fill the sclerosed acini and interspersed distorted myoepithelial cells remain *(Fig. 6.18.6)* 3. Glandular structures maintain a parallel or radial arrangement *(Fig. 6.18.7)*
Special studies	Myoepithelial cells not detected by immunohistochemistry	Immunohistochemistry for p63 highlights myoepithelial cells and emphasizes maintenance of lobulocentricity *(Fig. 6.18.8)*
Genetics	None to distinguish from DCIS	None to distinguish from invasive carcinoma
Treatment	Complete excision ± radiation, additional treatment based on receptor status and stage	Excision to negative margins ± radiation therapy; ± antiestrogen therapy
Clinical implication	Prognosis based on stage, grade, and receptor status	Risk of local recurrence as DCIS or invasive carcinoma if excision incomplete

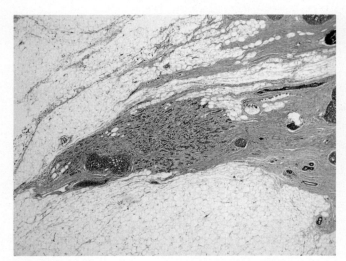

Figure 6.18.1   Invasive carcinoma of no special type: A small group of carcinoma cells mimics a large lobular unit, adjacent to expanded ducts.

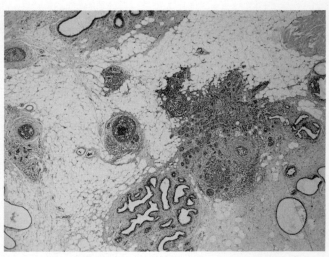

Figure 6.18.5   DCIS adjacent to and involving sclerosing adenosis. An irregular cluster of cells suggests an invasive process on low power.

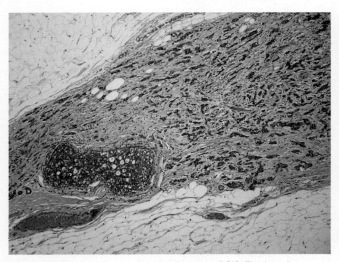

Figure 6.18.2   Invasive carcinoma adjacent to DCIS: The invasive component mimics lobulocentricity at low power and appears confined to stroma without infiltration into fat.

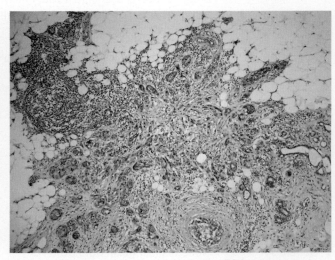

Figure 6.18.6   Sclerosing adenosis involved by DCIS: A lobulocentric arrangement is maintained, and neoplastic cells do not infiltrate fat.

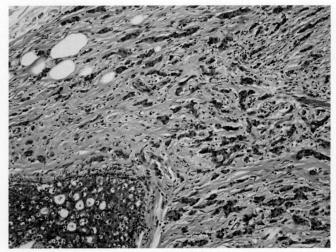

Figure 6.18.3   Invasive carcinoma adjacent to DCIS: The nests of invasive carcinoma are haphazardly arranged, infiltrating stroma and lacking a lobulocentric arrangement.

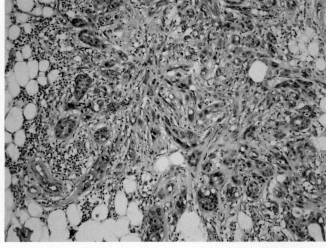

Figure 6.18.7   DCIS involving sclerosing adenosis: Characteristic findings suggesting the architecture of sclerosing adenosis include flattened spaces centrally that maintain a vaguely parallel arrangement, and more open spaces peripherally.

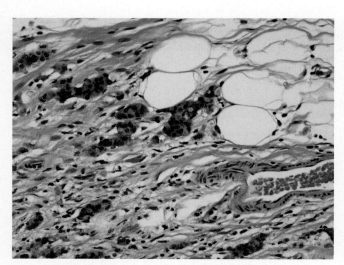

Figure 6.18.4   Fat infiltration by invasive carcinoma.

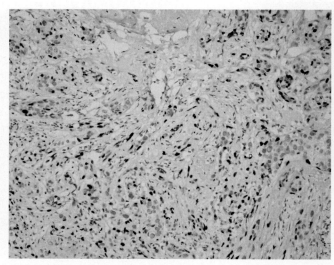

Figure 6.18.8   DCIS involving sclerosing adenosis: Myoepithelial cells are detected using immunohistochemistry for p63, supporting diagnosis of a noninvasive carcinoma.

	Low-Grade Invasive Mammary Carcinoma	Microglandular Adenosis
Age	Average age 60 y (usual range 45–75 y)	Most cases occur in 6th decade but age range wide (28–82 y)
Location	Anywhere in the breast	Anywhere in the breast
Presentation	Mammographic or palpable mass	Mammographic or palpable mass
Imaging findings	Nodular density, architectural distortion, or spiculated mass	No pathognomonic characteristics on mammography and ultrasound; 20%–50% present as architectural distortion or a mass lesion
Epidemiology	75%–80% of breast cancers diagnosed based on mammographic screening; 95% of palpable breast cancers; associated with family history, previous diagnosis of DCIS or atypical hyperplasia	Unknown
Histology	1. Haphazardly arranged glands, single cells, nests, islands, or cords of tumor *(Figs. 6.19.1–6.19.3)* 2. Cellular uniformity with low-grade nuclei *(Fig. 6.19.3)* 3. Myoepithelial layer lost throughout	1. Nonlobulocentric proliferation of uniform, small round glands irregularly infiltrating mammary stroma and adipose tissue *(Fig. 6.19.4)* 2. Glands composed of a single layer of cuboidal epithelial cells lacking apical snouts *(Fig. 6.19.5)* 3. Cells have clear cytoplasm and round nuclei with inconspicuous nucleoli *(Fig. 6.19.6)* 4. Glands surrounded by a basement membrane but lack a myoepithelial layer *(Fig. 6.19.6)* 5. Glands are not compressed by surrounding stroma. 6. Scattered glandular lumina contain secretions *(Fig. 6.19.6)*
Special studies	Usually strongly ER-positive; myoepithelial cells lacking using immunohistochemistry	PAS-positive, diastase resistant secretory material present in some lumina; strong immunoreactivity for S-100 protein, but lacks expression of myoepithelial markers or ER
Genetics	Grade I deletions 16q (>85%), gains 1q (60%), gains 16p (40%)	Recurrent losses of 5q and gains of 8q
Treatment	Complete excision, ± radiation, usually antiestrogen therapy, chemotherapy rarely indicated	None necessary when an incidental finding; excision to negative margins recommended for mass lesions
Clinical implication	Good to excellent prognosis in patients responsive to endocrine therapy	Benign process although large lesions may recur

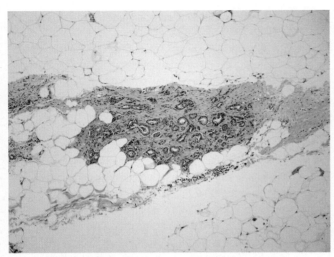

Figure 6.19.1 Small example of low-grade invasive mammary carcinoma with well-formed tubules.

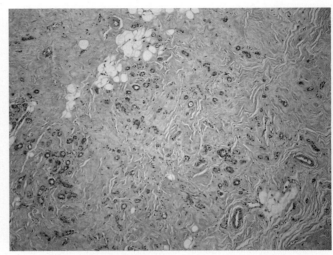

Figure 6.19.4 Microglandular adenosis: The stroma is diffusely infiltrated by cells arranged in round structures.

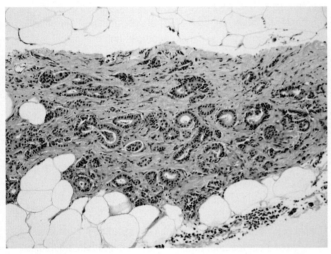

Figure 6.19.2 Invasive carcinoma of no special type composed of open and occasionally angulated tubules.

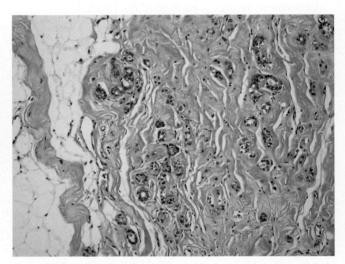

Figure 6.19.5 Microglandular adenosis: Open glandular structures lack a lobulocentric configuration.

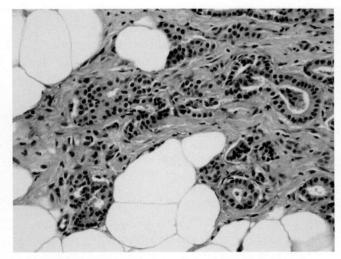

Figure 6.19.3 Invasive carcinoma composed of tubules and small nests having low-grade nuclei.

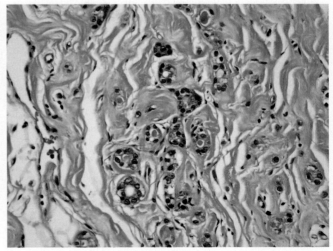

Figure 6.19.6 Microglandular adenosis composed of glands with a characteristic single cell lining, and central eosinophilic material.

SUGGESTED READINGS

Anderson TJ, Alexander FE, Forrest PM. The natural history of breast carcinoma: what have we learned from screening? *Cancer.* 2000;88:1758–1759.

Anderson TJ, Waller M, Ellis IO, et al. Influence of annual mammography from age 40 on breast cancer pathology. *Hum Pathol.* 2004;35:1252–1259.

Cabral AH, Recine M, Paramo JC, et al. Tubular carcinoma of the breast: an institutional experience and review of the literature. *Breast J.* 2003;9:298–301.

Dehner LP, Hill DA, Deschryver K. Pathology of the breast in children, adolescents, and young adults. *Semin Diagn Pathol.* 1999;16:235–247.

Diab SG, Clark GM, Osborne CK, et al. Tumor characteristics and clinical outcome of tubular and mucinous breast carcinomas. *J. Clin Oncol.* 1999;17:1442–1448.

Dixon JM, Anderson TJ, Page DL, et al. Infiltrating lobular carcinoma of the breast. *Histopathology.* 1982;6:149–161.

Dixon JM, Page DL, Anderson TJ, et al. Long-term survivors after breast cancer. *Br J Surg.* 1985;72:445–448.

Ellis IO, Galea M, Broughton N, et al. Pathological prognostic factors in breast cancer. II. Histological type. Relationship with survival in a large study with long-term follow-up. *Histopathology.* 1992;20:479–489.

Ellis IO, Schnitt SJ, Sastre-Garau X. Invasive breast carcinoma. In: Tavassoli FA, Devilee P, eds. *Tumours of the Breast and Female Genital Organs.* Lyon: IARC Press; 2003:13–59.

Farmer P, Bonnefoi H, Becette V, et al. Identification of molecular apocrine breast tumours by microarray analysis. *Oncogene.* 2005;24:4660–4671.

Farrow JH, Ashikari H. Breast lesions in young girls. *Surg Clin North Am.* 1969;49:261–269.

Geyer FC, Lacroix-Triki M, Colombo PE, et al. Molecular evidence in support of the neoplastic and precursor nature of microglandular adenosis. *Histopathology.* 2012;60:E115–E130.

Gobbi H, Simpson JF, Borowsky A, et al. Metaplastic breast tumors with a dominant fibromatosis-like phenotype have a high risk of local recurrence. *Cancer.* 1999;85:2170–2182.

Gobbi H, Simpson JF, Jensen RA, et al. Metaplastic spindle cell breast tumors arising within papillomas, complex sclerosing lesions, and nipple adenomas. *Mod Pathol.* 2003;16:893–901.

Horowitz DP, Sharma CS, Connolly E, et al. Secretory carcinoma of the breast: results from the survival, epidemiology and end results database. *Breast.* 2012;21:350–353.

Jacquemier J, Padovani L, Rabayrol L, et al. Typical medullary breast carcinomas have a basal/myoepithelial phenotype. *J Pathol.* 2005;207:260–268.

James BA, Cranor ML, Rosen PP. Carcinoma of the breast arising in microglandular adenosis. *Am J Clin Pathol.* 1993;100:507–513.

Japaze H, Emina J, Diaz C, et al. 'Pure' invasive apocrine carcinoma of the breast: a new clinicopathological entity? *Breast.* 2005;14:3–10.

Kasami M, Olson SJ, Simpson JF, et al. Maintenance of polarity and a dual cell population in adenoid cystic carcinoma of the breast: an immunohistochemical study. *Histopathology.* 1998;32:232–238.

Khalifeh IM, Albarracin C, Diaz LK, et al. Clinical, histopathologic, and immunohistochemical features of microglandular adenosis and transition into in situ and invasive carcinoma. *Am J Surg Pathol.* 2008;32:544–552.

Kitchen PR, Smith TH, Henderson MA, et al. Tubular carcinoma of the breast: prognosis and response to adjuvant systemic therapy. *ANZ J Surg.* 2001;71:27–31.

Krausz T, Jenkins D, Grontoft O, et al. Secretory carcinoma of the breast in adults: emphasis on late recurrence and metastasis. *Histopathology.* 1989;14:25–36.

Lae M, Freneaux P, Sastre-Garau X, et al. Secretory breast carcinomas with ETV6-NTRK3 fusion gene belong to the basal-like carcinoma spectrum. *Mod Pathol.* 2009;22:291–298.

Lee AK, Loda M, Mackarem G, et al. Lymph node negative invasive breast carcinoma 1 centimeter or less in size (T1a,bNOMO): clinicopathologic features and outcome. *Cancer.* 1997;79:761–771.

Lehmann BD, Bauer JA, Chen X, et al. Identification of human triple-negative breast cancer subtypes and preclinical models for selection of targeted therapies. *J Clin Invest.* 2011;121:2750–2767.

Louwman MW, Vriezen M, van Beek MW, et al. Uncommon breast tumors in perspective: incidence, treatment and survival in the Netherlands. *Int J Cancer.* 2007;121:127–135.

Masse SR, Rioux A, Beauchesne C. Juvenile carcinoma of the breast. *Hum Pathol.* 1981;12:1044–1046.

Mastropasqua MG, Maiorano E, Pruneri G, et al. Immunoreactivity for c-kit and p63 as an adjunct in the diagnosis of adenoid cystic carcinoma of the breast. *Mod Pathol.* 2005;18:1277–1282.

Nassar H, Wallis T, Andea A, et al. Clinicopathologic analysis of invasive micropapillary differentiation in breast carcinoma. *Mod Pathol.* 2001;14:836–841.

Oberman HA, Stephens PJ. Carcinoma of the breast in childhood. *Cancer.* 1972;30:470–474.

Page DL, Anderson TJ. *Diagnostic Histopathology of the Breast.* Edinburgh: Churchill Livingstone; 1987.

Page DL, Dixon JM, Anderson TJ, et al. Invasive cribriform carcinoma of the breast. *Histopathology.* 1983;7:525–536.

Page DL. Special types of invasive breast cancer, with clinical implications. *Am J Surg Pathol.* 2003;27:832–835.

Pastolero G, Hanna W, Zbieranowski I, et al. Proliferative activity and p53 expression in adenoid cystic carcinoma of the breast. *Mod Pathol.* 1996;9:215–219.

Paterakos M, Watkin WG, Edgerton SM, et al. Invasive micropapillary carcinoma of the breast: a prognostic study. *Hum Pathol.* 1999;30:1459–1463.

Pestalozzi BC, Zahrieh D, Mallon E, et al. Distinct clinical and prognostic features of infiltrating lobular carcinoma of the breast: combined results of 15 International Breast Cancer Study Group clinical trials. *J Clin Oncol.* 2008;26:3006–3014.

Prioleau PG, Santa Cruz DJ, Buettner JB, et al. Sweat gland differentiation in mammary adenoid cystic carcinoma. *Cancer.* 1979;43:1752–1760.

Rakha E, Pinder SE, Shin SJ, et al. Tubular carcinoma and cribriform carcinoma. In: Lakhani SR, Ellis, IO, Schnitt, SJ, et al., eds. *WHO Classification of Breast Tumors*. Lyon: IARC Press; 2012:43–45.

Rakha EA, El-Sayed ME, Menon S, et al. Histologic grading is an independent prognostic factor in invasive lobular carcinoma of the breast. *Breast Cancer Res Treat*. 2008;111:121–127.

Rakha EA, El-Sayed ME, Powe DG, et al. Invasive lobular carcinoma of the breast: response to hormonal therapy and outcomes. *Eur J Cancer*. 2008;44:73–83.

Rakha EA, Lee AH, Evans AJ, et al. Tubular carcinoma of the breast: further evidence to support its excellent prognosis. *J Clin Oncol*. 2010;28:99–104.

Resetkova E, Flanders DJ, Rosen PP. Ten-year follow-up of mammary carcinoma arising in microglandular adenosis treated with breast conservation. *Arch Pathol Lab Med*. 2003;127:77–80.

Ro JY, Silva EG, Gallager HS. Adenoid cystic carcinoma of the breast. *Hum Pathol*. 1987;18:1276–1281.

Sanders ME. Carcinomas with good prognosis. In: Palazzo J, ed. *Difficult Diagnoses in Breast Pathology*. New York: Demos; 2011:146.

Shin SJ, DeLellis RA, Ying L, et al. Small cell carcinoma of the breast: a clinicopathologic and immunohistochemical study of nine patients. *Am J Surg Pathol*. 2000;24:1231–1238.

Shin SJ, Rosen PP. Solid variant of mammary adenoid cystic carcinoma with basaloid features: a study of nine cases. *Am J Surg Pathol*. 2002;26:413–420.

Silverberg SG, Kay S, Chitale AR, et al. Colloid carcinoma of the breast. *Am J Clin Pathol*. 1971;55:355–363.

Simpson JF, Page DL. Prognostic value of histopathology in the breast. *Semin Oncol*. 1992;19:254–262.

Tanimura A, Konaka K. Carcinoma of the breast in a 5 years old girl. *Acta Pathol Jpn*. 1980;30:157–160.

Tavassoli F, Devilee P, eds. *Tumors of the Breast and Female Genital Organs*. 1st ed. Lyon: IRC Press; 2003.

Tavassoli FA, Norris HJ. Secretory carcinoma of the breast. *Cancer*. 1980;45:2404–2413.

Tognon C, Knezevich SR, Huntsman D, et al. Expression of the ETV6-NTRK3 gene fusion as a primary event in human secretory breast carcinoma. *Cancer Cell*. 2002;2:367–376.

Toikkanen S, Kujari H. Pure and mixed mucinous carcinomas of the breast: a clinicopathologic analysis of 61 cases with long-term follow-up. *Hum Pathol*. 1989;20:758–764.

Trendell-Smith NJ, Peston D, Shousha S. Adenoid cystic carcinoma of the breast: a tumour commonly devoid of oestrogen receptors and related proteins. *Histopathology*. 1999;35:241–248.

Venable JG, Schwartz AM, Silverberg SG. Infiltrating cribriform carcinoma of the breast: a distinctive clinicopathologic entity. *Hum Pathol*. 1990;21:333–338.

Vo TN, Meric-Bernstam F, Yi M, et al. Outcomes of breast-conservation therapy for invasive lobular carcinoma are equivalent to those for invasive ductal carcinoma. *Am J Surg*. 2006;192:552–555.

Walsh MM, Bleiweiss IJ. Invasive micropapillary carcinoma of the breast: eighty cases of an underrecognized entity. *Hum Pathol*. 2001;32:583–589.

Weigelt B, Baehner FL, Reis-Filho JS. The contribution of gene expression profiling to breast cancer classification, prognostication and prediction: a retrospective of the last decade. *J Pathol*. 2010;220:263–280.

Weigelt B, Horlings HM, Kreike B, et al. Refinement of breast cancer classification by molecular characterization of histological special types. *J Pathol*. 2008;216:141–150.

Wen YH, Weigelt B, Reis-Filho JS. Microglandular adenosis: a non-obligate precursor of triple-negative breast cancer? *Histol Histopathol*. 2013;28:1099–1108.

6 Invasive Carcinoma

7

Fibroepithelial Lesions

	Fibroadenoma	Hamartoma
Age	Any age, most frequent in women younger than 30 y old, frequently peri- and postpubertal adolescents	Any age, usually women in 4th or 5th decade
Presentation	Slow-growing, usually solitary, firm, mobile mass, typically less than 3 cm but may be larger	Soft palpable mass or asymptomatic, detected on imaging
Location	Anywhere in the breast or along the milk line	Anywhere in the breast
Imaging findings	Well-circumscribed, ovoid or multilobulated mass on mammogram; hypoechoic mass on ultrasound, wider than tall with distinct margins	Mammographically a well-circumscribed, round to oval mass containing fat and soft tissue with a thin, radiopaque pseudocapsule; by ultrasound, a circumscribed, round to oval mass, which may have intralesional heterogeneous echogenicity
Histology	1. Circumscribed, ovoid mass, smooth interface with surrounding mammary tissue, nonencapsulated *(Fig. 7.1.1)* 2. Ratio of stromal and glandular proliferation remains consistent throughout the lesion *(Fig. 7.1.2)* 3. Intracanalicular (glands compressed into cords by proliferating stroma) *(Fig. 7.1.3)* and pericanalicular (stroma surrounds epithelial elements with open lumina) patterns, admixed in most lesions; no clinical significance to patterns 3. Stroma uniform in cellularity and distribution, composed of mixture of collagen and bland, non-atypical stromal cells with ovoid nuclei *(Fig. 7.1.3)* 4. Rare stromal mitoses (less than 3 in 10 high-powered fields [HPF]) 5. The stroma may show a spectrum of changes, including multinucleated giant cells, myxoid change, PASH, hyalinization ± calcification, and rarely ossification 6. The epithelial component may show usual hyperplasia which is frequently mitotically active in adolescents, resembling gynecomastia	1. Lobulated mass incorporating normal mammary ducts, lobules and interlobular fibrous tissue within adipose tissue in varying proportions *(Fig. 7.1.4)* 2. Ducts and lobular units have a normal architectural arrangement *(Figs. 7.1.4 and 7.1.5)* 3. Demarcated from surrounding breast tissue by a thin, delicate capsule *(Fig. 7.1.4)* 4. Epithelial elements may show fibrocystic changes 5. Stroma may contain pseudoangiomatous stromal hyperplasia (PASH) or smooth muscle (myoid hamartoma) 6. Not easily diagnosed on core needle biopsy as complete architecture lacking
Special studies	None to distinguish from mammary hamartoma	Should be interpreted in radiologic context, which is usually defining

	Fibroadenoma	**Hamartoma**
Genetic abnormalities	Numerical abnormalities of chromosomes 16, 18, and 21; *MED12* and *RARA* mutations	May be seen in association with Cowden's syndrome. Aberrations involving 12q12-15 and 6p21 have been described.
Treatment	None required; may be excised for cosmesis if large or disfiguring	None necessary. Well-defined border/capsule usually allows for enucleation.
Clinical implication	Development of additional fibroadenomas	None. Rare local recurrences are of no consequence.

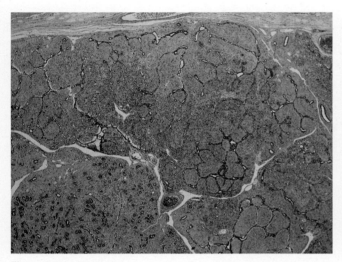

Figure 7.1.1 Fibroadenoma, showing sharp circumscription and a mixture of intracanalicular (top center) and pericanalicular (left lower) growth patterns.

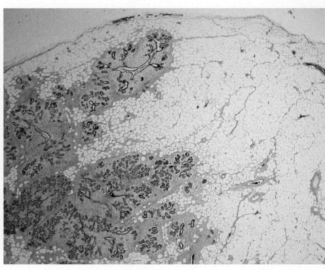

Figure 7.1.4 Hamartomas are well-circumscribed, lobulated masses containing architecturally normal lobular units and terminal ducts admixed with mature adipose tissue. Note the thin fibrous capsule (top).

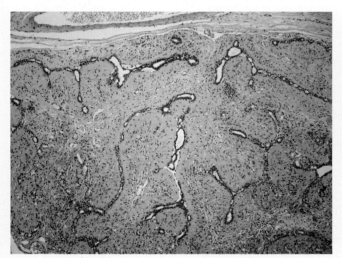

Figure 7.1.2 The interface of the fibroadenoma with the adjacent normal mammary parenchyma is sharply circumscribed. The epithelium is evenly distributed with respect to the stroma.

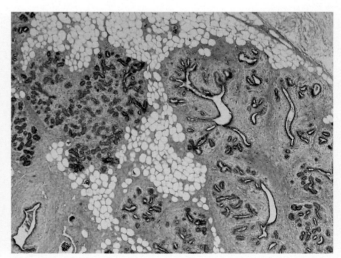

Figure 7.1.5 Segregation of the mature adipose tissue by encapsulation (upper right) is the defining feature of hamartoma.

7 Fibroepithelial Lesions

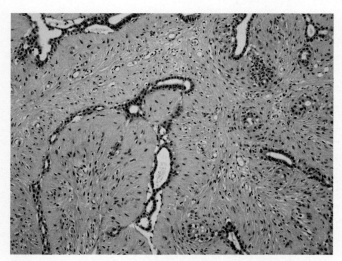

Figure 7.1.3   The epithelium is focally compressed by the collagenous stroma containing paucicellular bland spindle cells. The stromal nuclei are nonoverlapping, evenly distributed, and lack atypia.

	Fibroadenoma	Cellular Fibroadenoma
Age	Any age, most frequent in women younger than 30 y old; frequently peri- and postpubertal adolescents	Women younger than 30 y
Presentation	Slow-growing, solitary, mobile mass, typically less than 3 cm but may be larger; occasionally multiple and/or bilateral	Solitary, firm, palpable, mobile mass, typically less than 3 cm but may be larger; occasionally multiple and/or bilateral; may have history of rapid growth, otherwise no clinical findings to distinguish from ordinary fibroadenoma
Location	Anywhere in the breast or along the milk line	Anywhere in the breast or along the milk line
Imaging findings	Well-circumscribed, ovoid or multilobulated mass on mammogram; hypoechoic mass on ultrasound, wider than tall with distinct margins	Well-circumscribed, ovoid or multilobulated mass on mammogram; hypoechoic mass on ultrasound, wider than tall with distinct margins; no imaging findings to distinguish fibroadenoma from cellular fibroadenoma
Histology	1. Circumscribed, ovoid mass; smooth interface with surrounding mammary parenchyma; nonencapsulated *(Fig. 7.2.1)* 2. Proliferation of stromal and epithelial elements; ratio of stroma and glands remains relatively consistent throughout the lesion 3. Two patterns, intracanalicular (glands compressed into cords by proliferating stroma) and pericanalicular (stroma surrounds epithelial elements with open lumina), are admixed in most lesions; no clinical significance to patterns. Intracanalicular pattern may mimic benign phyllodes tumor *(Fig. 7.2.2)* 4. Stroma is uniform in cellularity and distribution, composed of a mixture of collagen and bland, non-atypical stromal cells with ovoid nuclei *(Fig. 7.2.3)* 5. Little mitotic activity ($<$3/HPF)	1. Circumscribed, ovoid mass, smooth interface with surrounding mammary tissue, nonencapsulated *(Fig. 7.2.4)* 2. Proliferation of stroma and epithelial elements; ratio of stroma and glands usually remains consistent throughout the lesion *(Fig. 7.2.4)*; both intracanalicular and pericanalicular patterns common 3. Increased stromal cellularity, but limited mitotic activity (usually $<$3/10 HPF) *(Figs. 7.2.5 and 7.2.6)* 4. Stromal cells lack atypia *(Fig. 7.2.6)*
Special studies	None to distinguish from cellular fibroadenoma	None to distinguish from ordinary fibroadenoma
Genetic abnormalities	Numerical abnormalities of chromosomes 16, 18, and 21; *MED12* and *RARA* mutations	Numerical abnormalities of chromosomes 16, 18, and 21; *MED12* and *RARA* mutations
Treatment	None required; may be excised for cosmesis if large or disfiguring	None required; may be excised for cosmesis if large or disfiguring

	Fibroadenoma	**Cellular Fibroadenoma**
Clinical implication	Development of additional fibroadenomas	The descriptors "giant" or "juvenile" fibroadenoma are clinical terms that describe rapid growth. The histologic correlate of these clinical terms is a cellular fibroadenoma that may show abundant hyperplasia that resembles gynectomastia. Mitotic activity in the epithelium and stroma (focally up to 5/10 HPF) is a result of hormonal stimulation and not an indication of aggressive clinical behavior.

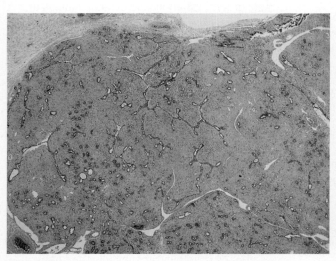

Figure 7.2.1   Fibroadenomas are nonencapsulated, stromal and epithelial proliferations that have a smooth interface with adjacent parenchyma.

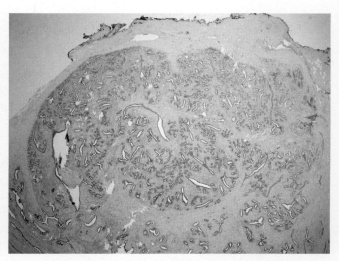

Figure 7.2.4   Cellular fibroadenoma showing a smooth interface with adjacent connective tissue. There are a few foci of intracanalicular growth lacking distortion.

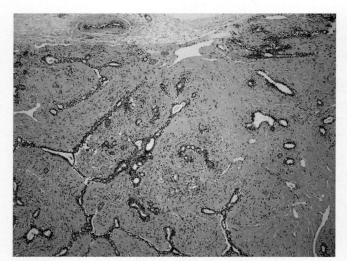

Figure 7.2.2   The epithelium is evenly distributed in a paucicellular stroma. The different epithelial patterns are of no clinical significance in a fibroadenoma, although an intracanalicular pattern (left) can occasionally mimic benign phyllodes tumor.

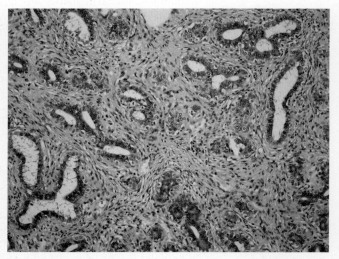

Figure 7.2.5   Stromal cellularity is increased but remains evenly distributed without stromal expansion in cellular fibroadenoma.

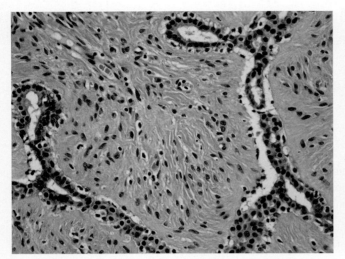

Figure 7.2.3   The stroma of this fibroadenoma is predominantly collagen, without increased stromal cellularity. The nuclei are bland and nonoverlapping.

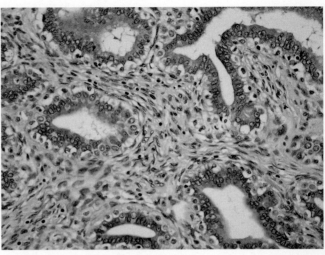

Figure 7.2.6   Cellular fibroadenoma, consisting of prominent stromal cells that lack atypia and mitotic activity. Myoepithelial cells are evident.

	Cellular Fibroadenoma	Benign Phyllodes Tumor
Age	Women younger than 30 y	Generally a decade older than women with fibroadenomas, occasionally younger women
Presentation	Solitary, firm, palpable, mobile mass, typically less than 3 cm but may be larger; occasionally multiple and/or bilateral; no clinical findings to distinguish from benign phyllodes tumor	Solitary, firm, palpable, mobile mass, frequently larger than 5 cm; very rarely multiple and/or bilateral; no clinical findings to distinguish from cellular fibroadenoma
Imaging findings	Well-circumscribed, ovoid or multilobulated mass on mammogram; hypoechoic mass on ultrasound, wider than tall with distinct margins; no imaging findings to consistently distinguish fibroadenoma from benign phyllodes tumor	Round, oval or lobulated, well-circumscribed mass on mammogram, may have a radiolucent halo; on ultrasound, inhomogeneous, solid mass containing cleft-like cystic spaces with posterior acoustic enhancement
Histology	1. Circumscribed, ovoid mass, smooth interface with surrounding mammary parenchyma, nonencapsulated *(Fig. 7.3.1)* 2. Proliferation of stroma and epithelial elements; ratio of stroma and glands usually remains consistent throughout the lesion *(Fig. 7.3.2)*; both intracanalicular and pericanalicular patterns common 3. Increased stromal cellularity, but limited mitotic activity (usually <3/10 HPF) *(Figs. 7.3.3–7.3.5)* 4. Stromal cells lack atypia *(Fig. 7.3.5)*	1. Circumscribed, lobulated proliferations of epithelium and expanded stroma, classically with a leaf-like architecture *(Figs. 7.3.6 and 7.3.7)* 2. The epithelium-bound leaf-like structures project into prominent epithelial-lined clefts formed by the expanded stroma *(Figs. 7.3.7 and 7.3.8)*. Epithelial distribution fairly regular throughout the lesion. 3. Stroma characterized by bland, spindled cells with mild atypia and mildly increased mitotic activity (usually <5/10 HPF) *(Figs. 7.3.9 and 7.3.10)*; stroma may be condensed around epithelial clefts. Stromal expansion may be uniform or heterogeneous. Stromal overgrowth absent 4. Squamous metaplasia common (rare in fibroadenoma) 5. Distinction between benign phyllodes tumor and cellular fibroadenoma may be difficult with the limited sample provided by core needle biopsy
Special studies	None to distinguish from benign phyllodes tumor	None to distinguish from fibroadenoma
Genetic abnormalities	Numerical abnormalities of chromosomes 16, 18, and 21; *MED12* and *RARA* mutations	Heterogeneous cytogenetic abnormalities. Mutations of *MED12* and *RARA*, *FLNA*, *SETD2*, and *KMT2D* reported.

	Cellular Fibroadenoma	**Benign Phyllodes Tumor**
Treatment	None required; may be excised for cosmesis if large or disfiguring	Excision; circumscription of benign phyllodes tumor may result in positive margin due "shelling-out." Clinical follow-up preferable to reexcision to maintain cosmesis.
Clinical implication	May develop additional fibroadenomas	Recurrence rates slightly higher than cellular fibroadenoma, approximately 10–15%

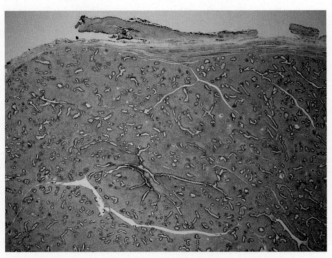

Figure 7.3.1 Cellular fibroadenoma has a smooth interface with the adjacent, compressed stroma. The epithelium is evenly distributed throughout the lesion.

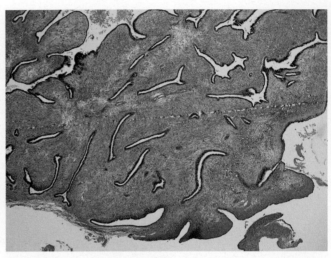

Figure 7.3.6 This benign phyllodes tumor is characterized by a prominent "leaf-like" pattern and cellular stroma, but the interface with the surrounding breast parenchyma remains smooth.

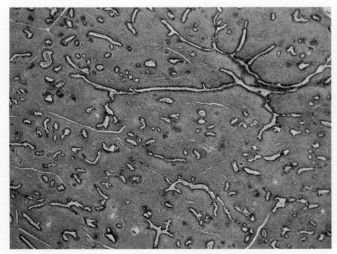

Figure 7.3.2 This cellular fibroadenoma has a focal intracanalicular growth pattern with elongated epithelial structures but lacks the distortion and degree of expansion required to qualify as a benign phyllodes tumor.

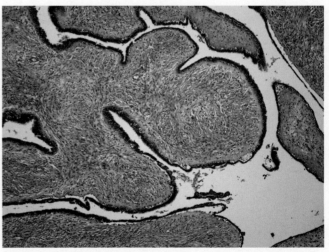

Figure 7.3.7 Nodules of proliferating stroma distort the epithelium in this benign phyllodes tumor.

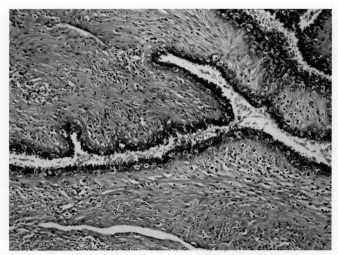

Figure 7.3.3   In cellular fibroadenoma, the stromal cellularity is mildly increased adjacent to elongated epithelial structures.

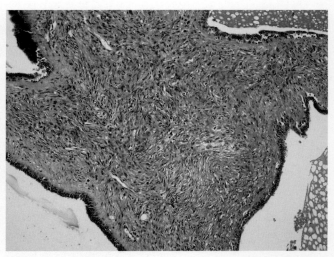

Figure 7.3.8   In benign phyllodes tumor, stromal cellularity is prominent.

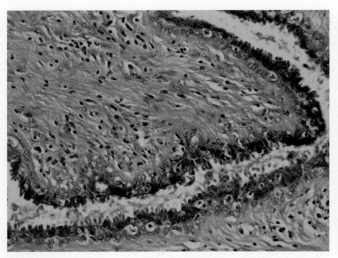

Figure 7.3.4   The bland spindled cells of this cellular fibroadenoma lack atypia and mitotic activity.

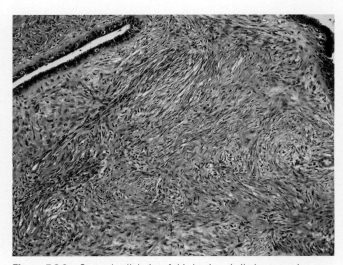

Figure 7.3.9   Stromal cellularity of this benign phyllodes tumor is pronounced but lacks atypia.

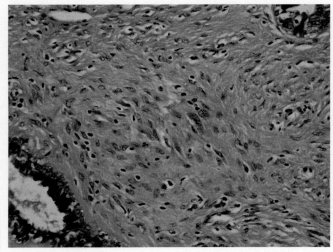

Figure 7.3.5   The stroma of cellular fibroadenoma may have focal myofibroblastic differentiation. There is no significant stromal atypia or mitotic activity.

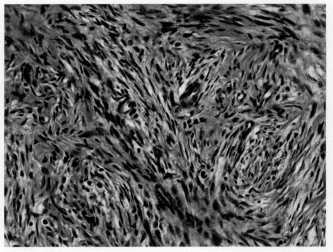

Figure 7.3.10   The stromal cells are crowded but lack significant atypia or mitotic activity.

	Benign Phyllodes Tumor	Borderline Phyllodes Tumor
Age	Women in 5th and 6th decades, occasionally younger women	Women in 5th and 6th decades, occasionally younger women
Presentation	Solitary, firm, palpable, mobile mass, frequently larger than 5 cm	Solitary, firm, palpable, mobile mass, frequently larger than 5 cm
Imaging findings	Round, oval or lobulated, well-circumscribed mass on mammogram, may have a radiolucent halo; on ultrasound, inhomogeneous, solid mass containing cleft-like cystic spaces with posterior acoustic enhancement	Round, oval or lobulated, well-circumscribed mass on mammogram, may have a radiolucent halo; on ultrasound, inhomogeneous, solid mass containing cleft-like cystic spaces with posterior acoustic enhancement; may have a more complex cystic echogenicity than benign phyllodes tumors
Histology	1. Circumscribed, lobulated proliferations of epithelium and expanded stroma, classically with a leaf-like architecture *(Figs. 7.4.1–7.4.2)* 2. The epithelium-bound leaf-like structures project into prominent epithelial-lined clefts, formed by the expanded stroma *(Fig. 7.4.2)*. Stroma may be condensed around epithelial clefts *(Fig. 7.4.2)*. Stromal expansion may be uniform or heterogeneous. Stromal overgrowth absent 4. Stroma characterized by bland to mildly atypical spindle cells and mildly increased mitotic activity (usually <5/10 HPF) *(Figs. 7.4.3–7.4.5)* 5. Squamous metaplasia common (rare in fibroadenoma) 6. Distinction between benign phyllodes tumor and borderline phyllodes tumor may be difficult with the limited sample provided by core needle biopsy	1. Fibroepithelial lesion composed of a cellular, expansile population of spindled cells showing mild to moderate nuclear atypia, distorting and compressing the accompanying bilayered epithelium, resulting in "leaf-like" structures *(Fig. 7.4.6)* 2. Frequently irregular interface with adjacent breast or adipose tissue *(Fig. 7.4.6)* including foci of permeative growth 3. Heterogeneously expanded stroma frequently results in uneven epithelial distribution *(Fig. 7.4.6)* 4. Stroma may be condensed around epithelial clefts *(Fig. 7.4.7)* 5. Frequent mitotic activity (5–10 mitoses/10 HPF) *(Figs. 7.4.8 and 7.4.9)* 6. Stromal expansion is prominent but does not meet formal definition of stromal overgrowth (4× field composed exclusively of stroma) 7. Limited foci suggesting low-grade fibrosarcoma may be seen
Special studies	None to distinguish among phyllodes tumor subtypes	None to distinguish among phyllodes tumor subtypes
Genetic abnormalities	Heterogeneous cytogenetic abnormalities. Mutations of *MED12*, *RARA*, *FLNA*, *SETD2*, and *KMT2D* reported.	Interstitial deletions of 9p21 (includes *CDKN2A* locus) and 9p. Mutations of *MED12*, *RARA*, *FLNA*, *SETD2*, and *KMT2D* reported.

	Benign Phyllodes Tumor	Borderline Phyllodes Tumor
Treatment	Excision; circumscription of benign phyllodes tumor may result in positive margin due "shelling-out." Clinical follow-up preferable to reexcision to maintain cosmesis	Excision with negative margins
Clinical implication	Recurrence rate of approximately 10–15%	Recurrence rates higher than benign phyllodes tumor, approximately 20%

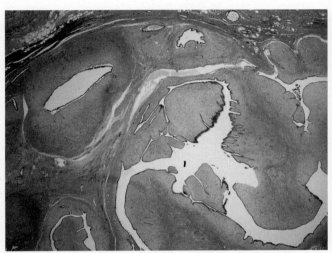

Figure 7.4.1   This benign phyllodes tumor is circumscribed with prominent "leaf-like" epithelial structures formed by the expanded stroma. Stromal condensation adjacent to the epithelium is a frequent finding.

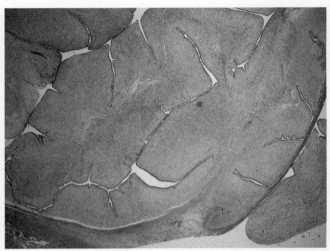

Figure 7.4.6   Borderline phyllodes tumor showing stromal expansion, distorted "leaf-like" epithelium, and irregular borders.

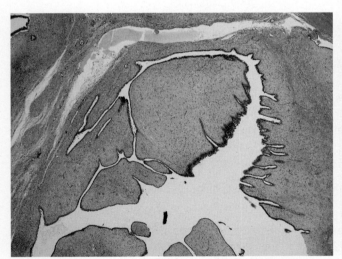

Figure 7.4.2   The expanded stroma distorts the associated epithelium, resulting in prominent epithelial-lined clefts and leaf-like projections.

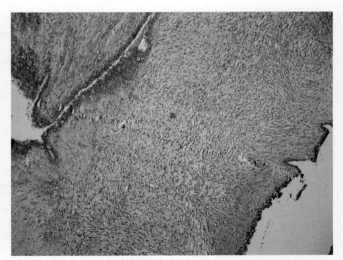

Figure 7.4.7   The cellular stroma is condensed adjacent to the epithelium in this borderline phyllodes tumor.

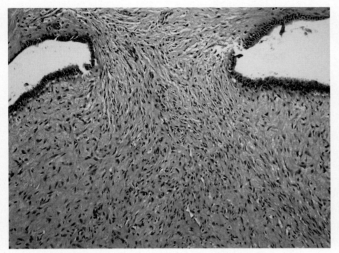

Figure 7.4.3 Moderate stromal cellularity and mild nuclear atypia characterize benign phyllodes tumor.

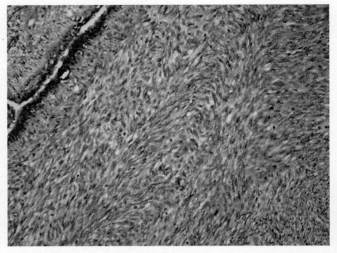

Figure 7.4.8 The stroma is quite cellular and expanded but does not meet the definition of stromal "overgrowth" (4× field devoid of epithelium) in this borderline phyllodes tumor.

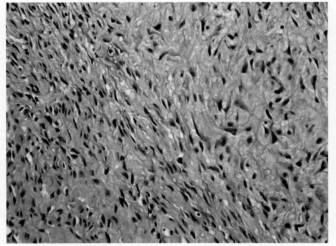

Figure 7.4.4 Although the stroma is cellular in benign phyllodes tumor, abundant collagen remains. Stromal cells are spindled with only mild atypia. Some mitotic activity is expected but as a single criterion does not upgrade the phyllodes tumor category in the absence of other features (see borderline phyllodes tumor).

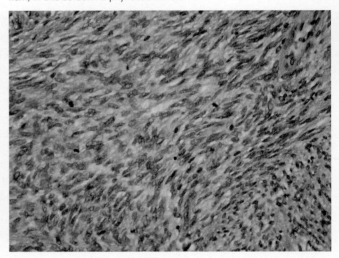

Figure 7.4.9 Mitotic activity and moderate stromal atypia are evident in this borderline phyllodes tumor.

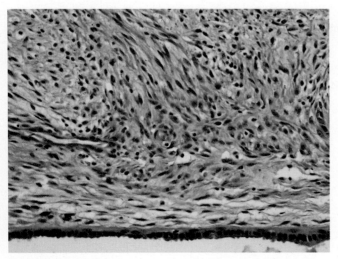

Figure 7.4.5 Often the stromal proliferation is more pronounced adjacent to the epithelium, forming the so called "cambium layer."

	Borderline Phyllodes Tumor	Malignant Phyllodes Tumor
Age	Women in 5th and 6th decades	Women in 5th and 6th decades, or older
Presentation	Solitary, firm, palpable, mobile mass, frequently larger than 5 cm	Solitary, firm, palpable, mobile mass, frequently larger than 5 cm
Imaging findings	Round, oval or lobulated, well-circumscribed mass on mammogram, may have a radiolucent halo; on ultrasound, inhomogeneous, solid mass containing cleft-like cystic spaces with posterior acoustic enhancement; may have more complex cystic echogenicity than benign phyllodes tumor	Round, oval or lobulated, well-circumscribed mass on mammogram, may have a radiolucent halo; on ultrasound, inhomogeneous, solid mass containing cleft-like cystic spaces with posterior acoustic enhancement; typically more complex cystic echogenicity than border-line phyllodes tumor
Histology	1. Cellular, expansile population of spindled cells showing mild to moderate nuclear atypia, distorting and compressing an accompanying bilayered epithelium, resulting in "leaf-like" structures *(Figs. 7.5.1 and 7.5.2)*. Stroma may be condensed around epithelial clefts 2. Frequently irregular interface with adjacent breast or adipose tissue *(Fig. 7.5.3)*, including foci of permeative growth 3. Heterogeneously expanded stroma results in uneven epithelial distribution *(Fig. 7.5.1)* 4. Frequent mitotic activity (5–10 mitoses/10 HPF) *(Fig. 7.5.4)* 5. Stromal expansion is prominent but does not meet the formal definition of stromal overgrowth (4× field composed exclusively of stroma) *(Fig. 7.5.1)* 6. Limited foci suggesting low-grade fibrosarcoma may be seen	1. Moderate to marked stromal cellularity and atypia with frequent mitoses (>10 mitoses/10 HPF) *(Figs. 7.5.5–7.5.8)*. Classic leaf-like architecture may not be evident 2. Stromal cellularity and distribution frequently heterogeneous with sarcomatous stromal overgrowth defining for malignant phyllodes (4× field composed exclusively of stroma). Overgrowth may be regional, highlighting the importance of adequate sampling *(Fig. 7.5.6)* 3. Sarcoma component may be low, intermediate, or high grade *(Figs. 7.5.7 and 7.5.8)* 4. May have heterologous sarcomatous differentiation 5. Irregular to infiltrative interface with surrounding parenchyma frequent *(Fig. 7.5.6)* 6. The above features are commonly, but not always, present in combination
Special studies	None to distinguish among phyllodes tumor subtypes	None to distinguish among phyllodes tumor subtypes
Genetic abnormalities	Interstitial deletions of 9p21 (includes *CDKN2A* locus) and 9p. Mutations of *MED12, RARA, FLNA, SETD2,* and *KMT2D* reported.	Extensive cytogenetic abnormalities that increase in number with tumor grade, including gains on chromosome 1q and losses on chromosome 13 which are reported to be associated with malignant progression. Interstitial deletions of 9p21 (includes *CDKN2A* locus) and 9p. Mutations of *MED12, RARA, FLNA, SETD2,* and *KMT2D* reported.

	Borderline Phyllodes Tumor	**Malignant Phyllodes Tumor**
Treatment	Excision with negative margins	Excision with negative margins
Clinical implication	Recurrence rates of approximately 20%	Low-grade malignant phyllodes tumors have capacity for local recurrence only; intermediate- and high-grade malignant phyllodes tumors may metastasize, although uncommonly

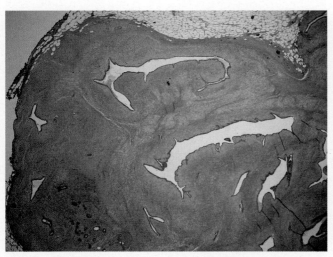

Figure 7.5.1   The interface with the surrounding adipose tissue is characteristically irregular in borderline phyllodes tumors. The epithelial clefts are distorted by cellular stroma.

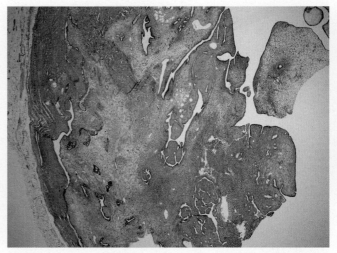

Figure 7.5.5   Heterogeneous stromal expansion and high cellularity evident on low power readily identify this lesion as a malignant phyllodes tumor. A leaf-like growth pattern is maintained in the majority of the lesion.

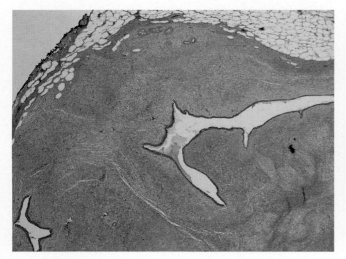

Figure 7.5.2   Although the stroma is markedly cellular, a 4× field devoid of epithelium is absent, hence the borderline designation for this phyllodes tumor.

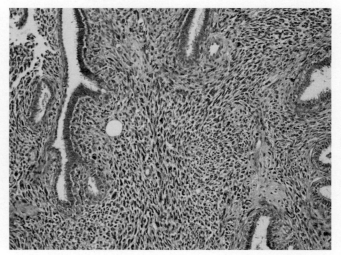

Figure 7.5.6   Malignant phyllodes tumor: Although some glandular elements are evident in any given 4× field, the stroma is markedly cellular and atypical with high mitotic activity requiring a diagnosis of malignant phyllodes tumor.

7 Fibroepithelial Lesions

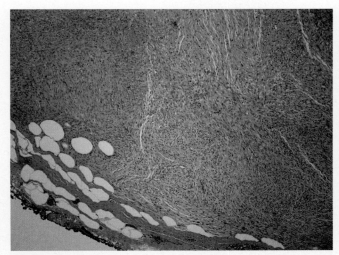

Figure 7.5.3 A borderline phyllodes tumor showing permeative growth into fat.

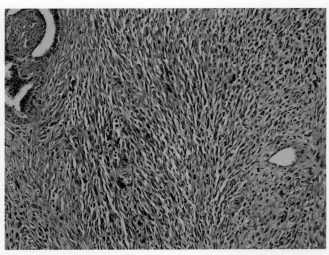

Figure 7.5.7 In this malignant phyllodes tumor the stroma is densely cellular, with a herringbone pattern, composed of spindled cells with hyperchromatic nuclei.

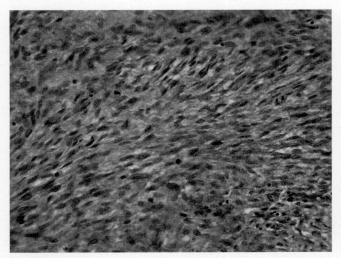

Figure 7.5.4 A borderline phyllodes tumor showing mitotic activity and moderate stromal atypia.

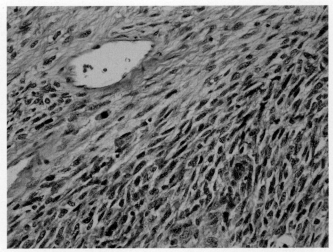

Figure 7.5.8 Marked nuclear pleomorphism is evident, as well as numerous mitotic figures, including abnormal mitoses in this malignant phyllodes tumor.

	Malignant Phyllodes Tumor	Primary Sarcoma
Age	Women in 5th and 6th decades, or older, rarely young women	Women in 5th and 6th decades, or older
Presentation	Solitary, firm, palpable, mobile mass, frequently larger than 5 cm	Solitary, firm, palpable, fixed mass, frequently larger than 5 cm
Imaging findings	Lobulated, well- to poorly-circumscribed mass on mammogram, may have a radiolucent halo; on ultrasound, inhomogeneous, solid mass containing cleft-like cystic spaces with posterior acoustic enhancement; typically complex cystic echogenicity	Irregular to spiculated mass, taller than wide with indistinct margins; lacks cleft-like cystic spaces
Histology	1. Stromal cellularity and distribution frequently heterogeneous *(Fig. 7.6.1)*; sarcomatous stromal overgrowth *(Fig. 7.6.2)* defining for malignant phyllodes (4× field composed exclusively of stroma). Overgrowth may be regional, highlighting the importance of adequate sampling 2. Foci diagnostic of high-grade sarcoma with marked stromal cellularity, marked atypia, and frequent mitoses (>10 mitoses/10 HPF) may be focal *(Figs. 7.6.3–7.6.5)* 3. To distinguish from pure sarcoma, an epithelial component must be identified at least focally, although the classic leaf-like architecture may not be present *(Fig. 7.6.1)* 4. Heterologous sarcomatous differentiation may complicate distinction from primary sarcoma when the epithelial component is focal. 5. Irregular interface with infiltrative growth into the surrounding parenchyma frequent *(Fig. 7.6.1)* 6. Above features are commonly but not always present in combination	1. Expansile growth of malignant spindled cells *(Fig. 7.6.5)* 2. No epithelial elements present *(Figs. 7.6.5 and 7.6.6)* 3. Marked pleomorphism with frequent mitotic figures *(Figs. 7.6.7–7.6.8)*
Special studies	None to definitively distinguish from primary sarcoma; cytokeratin staining may highlight pattern of epithelial component, helping to distinguish from infiltration among neighboring epithelial elements	Negative for markers of epithelial, vascular, or melanocytic differentiation
Genetic abnormalities	Extensive cytogenetic abnormalities which increase in number with tumor grade, including gains on chromosome 1q and losses on chromosome 13 which are reported to be associated with malignant progression. Interstitial deletions of 9p21 (includes *CDKN2A* locus) and 9p. Mutations of *MED12, RARA, FLNA, SETD2,* and *KMT2D* reported.	Multiple complex abnormalities which increase in number with tumor grade

	Malignant Phyllodes Tumor	**Primary Sarcoma**
Treatment	Excision with negative margins	Excision with negative margins
Clinical implication	Low-grade malignant phyllodes tumors have capacity for local recurrence only; intermediate- or high-grade malignant phyllodes tumors less likely to metastasize than primary sarcoma	High propensity for systemic metastasis

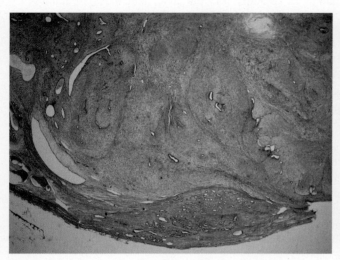

Figure 7.6.1   This malignant phyllodes tumor shows stromal overgrowth with distortion of the limited remaining epithelial component.

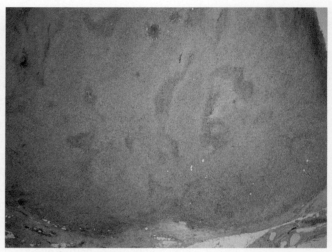

Figure 7.6.5   Primary breast sarcoma: Expansile mass consisting of malignant spindled cells without epithelial elements.

Figure 7.6.2   Stromal overgrowth in this malignant phyllodes tumor as defined by a 4× field devoid of epithelial elements.

Figure 7.6.6   Malignant spindled cells lacking obvious differentiation. No epithelial elements are present within this primary breast sarcoma.

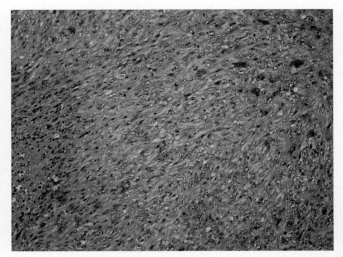

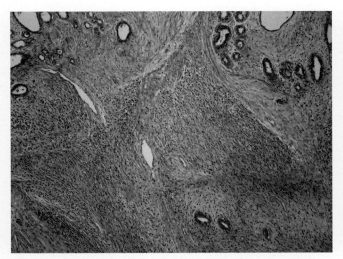

Figure 7.6.3   In another region, a few distorted glandular structures are associated with markedly cellular stroma in this malignant phyllodes tumor.

Figure 7.6.7   Primary sarcomas commonly contain areas of geographic necrosis (left lower).

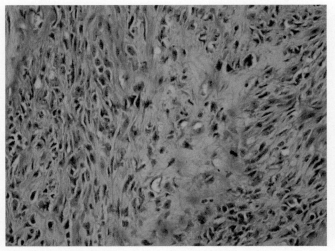

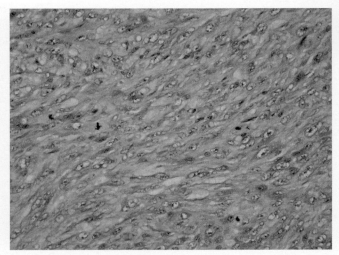

Figure 7.6.4   Malignant phyllodes tumor with pleomorphic spindled cells and mitotic figures.

Figure 7.6.8   Primary breast sarcoma characterized by markedly pleomorphic spindled cells showing numerous mitoses.

SUGGESTED READINGS

Bernstein L, Deapen D, Ross RK. The descriptive epidemiology of malignant cystosarcoma phyllodes tumors of the breast. *Cancer.* 1993;71:3020–3024.

Carter BA, Page DL, Schuyler P, et al. No elevation in long-term breast carcinoma risk for women with fibroadenomas that contain atypical hyperplasia. *Cancer.* 2001;92:30–36.

Chang HL, Lerwill MF, Goldstein AM. Breast hamartomas in adolescent females. *Breast J.* 2009;15:515–520.

Chen WH, Cheng SP, Tzen CY, et al. Surgical treatment of phyllodes tumors of the breast: retrospective review of 172 cases. *J Surg Oncol.* 2005;91:185–194.

Cohn-Cedermark G, Rutqvist LE, Rosendahl I, et al. Prognostic factors in cystosarcoma phyllodes. A clinicopathologic study of 77 patients. *Cancer.* 1991;68:2017–2022.

Cowan ML, Argani P, Cimino-Matthews A. Benign and low grade fibroepithelial neoplasms of the breast have a low recurrence rate after positive surgical margins. *Mod Pathol.* 2016; 29(3):259–265.

Daya D, Trus T, D'Souza TJ, et al. Hamartoma of the breast, an underrecognized breast lesion. A clinicopathologic and radiographic study of 25 cases. *Am J Clin Pathol.* 1995;103:685–689.

Dupont WD, Page DL, Parl FF, et al. Long-term risk of breast cancer in women with fibroadenoma. *N Engl J Med.* 1994;331:10–15.

Grady I, Gorsuch H, Wilburn-Bailey S. Long-term outcome of benign fibroadenomas treated by ultrasound-guided percutaneous excision. *Breast J.* 2008;14:275–278.

Hawkins RE, Schofield JB, Fisher C, et al. The clinical and histologic criteria that predict metastases from cystosarcoma phyllodes. *Cancer.* 1992;69:141–147.

Jacobs TW, Chen YY, Guinee DG Jr, et al. Fibroepithelial lesions with cellular stroma on breast core needle biopsy: are there predictors of outcome on surgical excision? *Am J Clin Pathol.* 2005;124:342–354.

Lakhani SR, Ellis IO, Schnitt SJ, et al., eds. *WHO Classification of Tumors of the Breast.* 4 ed. Lyon: IARC; 2012.

Linell F, Ostberg G, Soderstrom J, et al. Breast hamartomas. An important entity in mammary pathology. *Virchows Arch A Pathol Anat Histol.* 1979;383:253–264.

Moffat CJ, Pinder SE, Dixon AR, et al. Phyllodes tumours of the breast: a clinicopathological review of thirty-two cases. *Histopathology.* 1995;27:205–218.

Mollitt DL, Golladay ES, Gloster ES, et al. Cystosarcoma phylloides in the adolescent female. *J Pediatr Surg.* 1987;22:907–910.

Sanders M, Boulos F. The Breast. In: Gilbert-Barness E, ed. *Potter's Pathology of the Fetus, Infant and Child.* 2nd ed. Philadelphia: Mosby Elsevier; 2007:2093–2114.

Tan PH, Jayabaskar T, Chuah KL, et al. Phyllodes tumors of the breast: the role of pathologic parameters. *Am J Clin Pathol.* 2005;123:529–540.

Tan PH, Thike AA, Tan WJ, et al. Predicting clinical behaviour of breast phyllodes tumours: a nomogram based on histological criteria and surgical margins. *J Clin Pathol.* 2012;65:69–76.

Tan PH, Tse G, Lee A, et al. Fibroepithelial tumors. In: Lakhani SR, Ellis IO, Schnitt SJ, et al., eds. *WHO Classification of Tumor of the Breast.* Lyon: IARC; 2012:141–147.

Tse GM, Law BK, Ma TK, et al. Hamartoma of the breast: a clinicopathological review. *J Clin Pathol.* 2002;55:951–954.

8

Benign and Reactive Stromal Lesions

	Pseudoangiomatous Stromal Hyperplasia (PASH)	Stromal Fibrosis
Age	Any age, usually premenopausal women, association with contraceptive use; postmenopausal women on hormone therapy; men with gynecomastia	Adolescents and premenopausal women
Location	Anywhere in the breast	Anywhere in the breast
Presentation	Clinical mass or incidental finding	Clinical mass or incidental finding
Imaging findings	Mammographic mass without calcification; on ultrasound, a well-defined hypoechoic mass; MRI may show non–mass-like enhancement	None or parenchymal distortion
Etiology	Hormone imbalance, aberrant response to hormones	Unknown
Histology	1. Myofibroblastic proliferation usually well demarcated *(Fig. 8.1.1)* 2. Myofibroblasts form slit-shaped, pseudovascular spaces devoid of red blood cells within a dense, keloid-like stroma *(Figs. 8.1.2 and 8.1.3)*	1. Periductal and perilobular fibrosis, may form a discrete mass *(Fig. 8.1.4)* 2. Fibrosis consists of dense collagen of low cellularity *(Fig. 8.1.5)* 3. Associated epithelial elements often atrophic *(Fig. 8.1.4)* 4. Occasional true vascular spaces (capillaries and lymphatic spaces) are present *(Fig. 8.1.6)*
Special studies	None routinely needed. The cells lining the pseudovascular spaces express vimentin and CD34, and are negative for Factor VIII and CD31.	None
Genetic abnormalities	None	None
Treatment	PASH is a benign process which requires excision only for cosmesis and to eliminate discomfort	None
Clinical implication	None	None

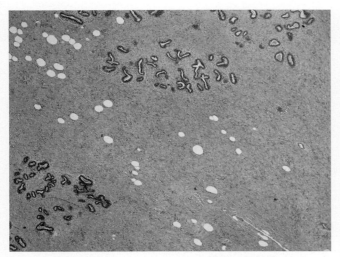

Figure 8.1.1   PASH is composed of bland, densely fibrotic stroma replacing interlobular and specialized intralobular connective tissue.

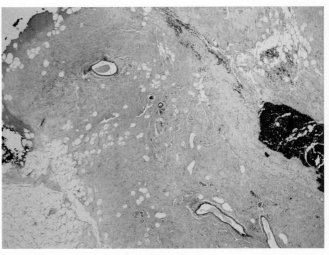

Figure 8.1.4   Periductal and perilobular fibrosis consists of expansile dense collagen, often concentrically arranged around atrophic epithelial elements with or without formation of a discrete mass.

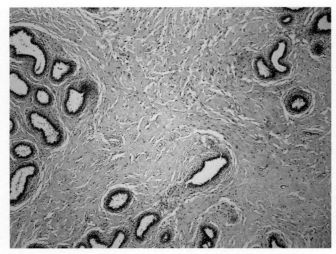

Figure 8.1.2   The myofibroblasts impart a keloidal appearance and are interposed among the preexisting epithelial elements without deforming them.

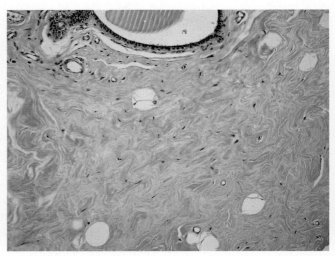

Figure 8.1.5   The fibrosis consist of delicate bands of wavy, eosinophilic, nearly acellular collagen.

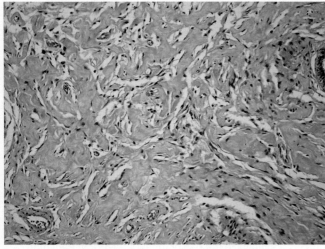

Figure 8.1.3   The myofibroblastic proliferation in PASH forms slit-shaped, pseudovascular spaces devoid of red blood cells.

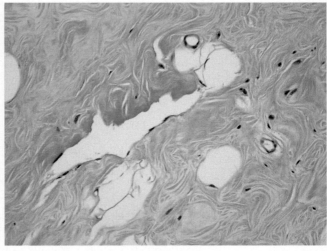

Figure 8.1.6   Occasional true vascular spaces are present.

8 Stromal Lesions

	Nodular Fasciitis	Fibromatosis
Age	Adult women, occasionally occurs in men, wide age range	Wide age range, more common in women but may occur in men
Location	Subcutis of the breast or less commonly within the mammary parenchyma	Most frequently arises from the pectoral fascia and extends into the breast but may occasionally originate within the breast parenchyma
Presentation	Mass; history of rapid growth and tenderness	Single nontender palpable mass; may be accompanied by skin retraction or dimpling; rarely bilateral
Imaging findings	Mass, frequently with infiltrative margins mammographically. On ultrasound, homogeneous, hypoechoic, solid mass with a border often obscured by normal tissues.	Spiculated mass
Etiology	Usually history of trauma, although eliciting that history may be difficult	Unknown; may be associated with previous trauma, surgery, and breast implants
Histology	1. Dense, nodular, well-circumscribed proliferation of myofibroblasts lacking a capsule (Fig. 8.2.1) 2. Plump fibroblastic and myofibroblastic cells arranged in short fascicles in edematous stroma (Fig. 8.2.2) 3. Hemorrhage common (Fig. 8.2.3) 4. Edematous, occasionally myxoid stroma, containing lymphocytes, erythrocytes, and thin-walled vessels; stromal changes often described as "tissue culture" fibroblastic proliferation (Figs. 8.2.3 and 8.2.4) 5. Mitoses and osteoclast-like giant cells may be present	1. Poorly circumscribed mass (Fig. 8.2.5) 2. Locally infiltrative stromal neoplasm composed of long sweeping, intersecting fascicles of bland fibroblasts and myofibroblasts (Figs. 8.2.6 and 8.2.7) 3. Variable cellularity, with the more cellular regions usually present at the periphery (Fig. 8.2.5) 4. Perivascular hemorrhage; no (or rare) mitotic figures 5. Dense collagen resembles a keloid (Fig. 8.2.7) 6. Irregular "tongues" of cellular stroma extend into fat (Figs. 8.2.5, 8.2.6, and 8.2.8)
Special studies	Expresses the muscle marker actin; desmin positivity rare. Keratin, S100, and CD34 usually negative.	Cytoplasmic expression of actin and nuclear expression of β-catenin in 80% of cases. Desmin and S-100 expression may be detected in a minority of cells. Fibromatosis is negative for expression of cytokeratins, BCL-2, CD34, estrogen (ER), progesterone (PR), and androgen receptors (AR).
Genetic abnormalities	Recurrent MYH9-USP6 gene fusions	May arise in patients with familial adenomatous polyposis coli (FAP), but most are sporadic. Activating mutations in β-catenin gene reported in 45% of cases, mutations in FAP or 5q loss reported in 33% of cases.
Treatment	None. When characteristic histologic features are present in the appropriate clinical setting, observation is sufficient, with the expectation that the mass will eventually resolve.	If anatomically feasible, wide local excision to obtain negative margins should be undertaken to minimize the risk of local recurrence. Radiation and chemotherapy ineffective and not indicated.

	Nodular Fasciitis	**Fibromatosis**
Clinical implication	None. Local recurrence infrequent.	Local recurrence in 20%–30% of cases, usually within 3 y of original diagnosis; lacks metastatic potential

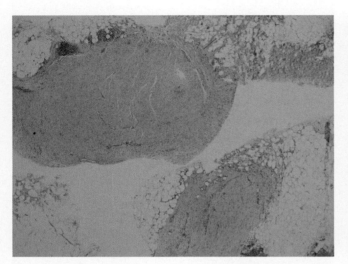

Figure 8.2.1   Nodular fasciitis lacks a capsule but is well circumscribed.

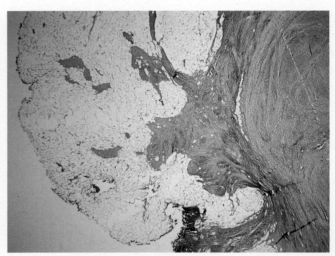

Figure 8.2.5   The irregular fibroblastic proliferation of fibromatosis extends into adjacent fat.

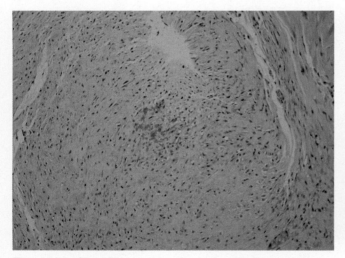

Figure 8.2.2   Plump fibroblastic/myofibrolastic cells with pale eosinophilic cytoplasm arranged in short fascicles characterize nodular fasciitis.

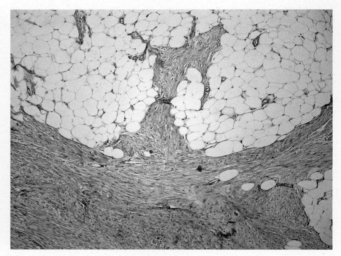

Figure 8.2.6   Fibromatosis often shows irregular "tongues" of fibroblastic cells extending into fat.

8 Stromal Lesions

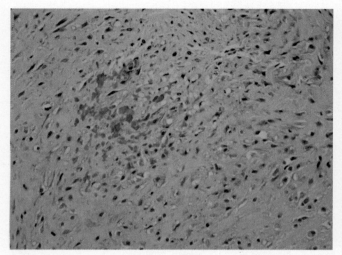

Figure 8.2.3   The stroma of nodular fasciitis is edematous and occasionally myxoid with lymphocytes, extravasated erythrocytes, and thin-walled vessels.

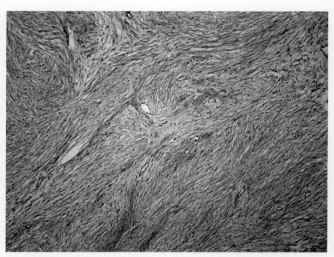

Figure 8.2.7   Broad sweeping fascicles of fibroblastic cells have interspersed keloidal type collagen.

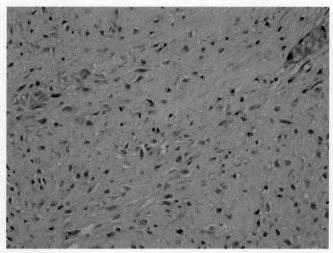

Figure 8.2.4   The stromal changes of nodular fasciitis are often described as a "tissue culture-like" fibroblastic proliferation. Mitoses may be present.

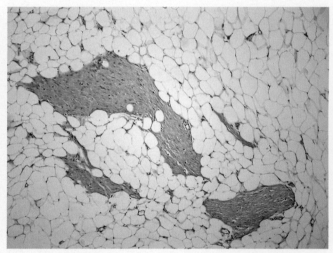

Figure 8.2.8   Insidious permeation of surrounding tissues may lead to incomplete excision and local recurrence.

	Fibromatosis	Scar
Age	Wide age range, more common in females	Middle age to older women
Location	Most frequently arises from the pectoral fascia and extends into the breast but may occasionally originate within the breast parenchyma	Prior surgical or trauma site, near implants
Presentation	Single, nontender, palpable mass; may be accompanied by skin retraction or dimpling; rarely bilateral	History of prior breast biopsy/surgery, including implants
Imaging findings	Spiculated mass	Architectural distortion, dystrophic calcifications, and asymmetry
Etiology	Unknown; may be associated with previous trauma, surgery, and breast implants	Prior breast biopsy/surgery, including implants, ruptured cyst, resolving fat necrosis
Histology	1. Poorly circumscribed mass *(Fig. 8.3.1)* 2. Locally infiltrative stromal neoplasm, composed of long sweeping, intersecting fascicles of bland fibroblasts and myofibroblasts *(Figs. 8.3.2 and 8.3.3)* 3. Variable cellularity, with the more cellular regions usually present at the periphery 4. Pericapillary hemorrhage; no (or rare) mitotic figures 5. May invade into normal structures	1. Composed of dense collagen containing sparse fibroblasts *(Fig. 8.3.4)* 2. Interspersed foamy macrophages, foreign body giant cells, foci of fat necrosis, hemosiderin-laden macrophages, and neovascularization *(Figs. 8.3.5 and 8.3.6)*
Special studies	Cytoplasmic expression of actin and nuclear expression of β-catenin in 80% of cases. Desmin and S-100 expression may be detected in a minority of cells. Fibromatosis is negative for expression of cytokeratins, BCL-2, CD34, ER, PR, and AR.	Lacks nuclear β-catenin expression
Genetic abnormalities	May arise in patients with *FAP*, but most are sporadic. Activating mutations in β-catenin gene reported in 45% of cases; mutations in *FAP* or 5q loss reported in 33% of cases.	None
Treatment	If anatomically feasible, wide local excision to obtain negative margins should be undertaken to minimize the risk of local recurrence. Radiation and chemotherapy ineffective and thus not indicated.	None, excision for cosmesis only
Clinical implication	Local recurrence in 20%–30% of cases, usually within 3 y of original diagnosis; lacks metastatic potential	None

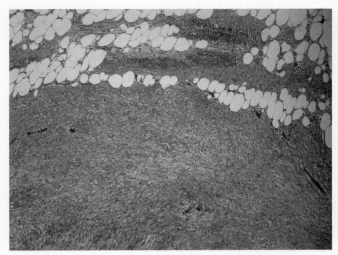

Figure 8.3.1   Fibromatosis characterized by a poorly circumscribed proliferation of fibroblastic cells with irregular "'tongues" extending into fat.

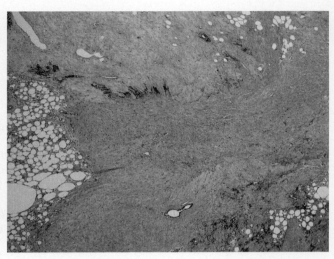

Figure 8.3.4   Scar juxtaposed to dense stromal fibrosis and fat necrosis.

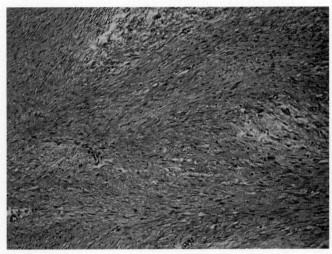

Figure 8.3.2   Fibromatosis with characteristic broad sweeping fascicles of fibroblasts with variably edematous stroma.

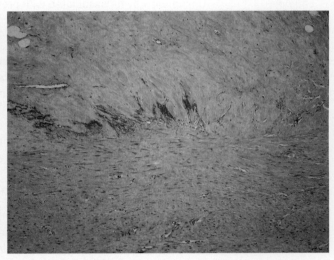

Figure 8.3.5   The fibrosis of a scar is paucicellular in comparison to fibromatosis (Figs. 8.3.2 and 8.3.3).

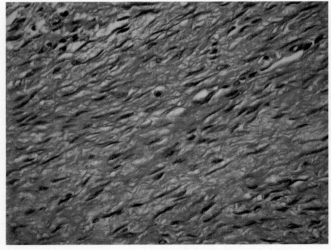

Figure 8.3.3   Fibroblasts and myofibroblasts have elongated, often "wavy," nuclei. Mitotic activity is absent or rare.

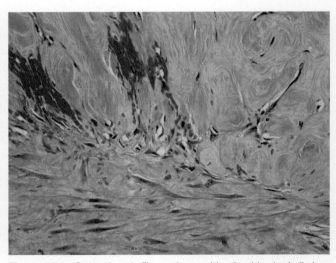

Figure 8.3.6   Predominantly fibrous tissue with a few bland spindled fibroblasts and neovessels characterizes scar.

	Fibromatosis	Fibromatosis-like Metaplastic Carcinoma
Age	Wide age range, more common in females than males	Middle age women 50–70 y, similar to age range of invasive carcinomas of no special type
Location	Most frequently arises from the pectoral fascia and extends into the breast, but may occasionally originate within the breast parenchyma	Anywhere in the breast
Presentation	Single, nontender, palpable mass; may be accompanied by skin retraction or dimpling; rarely bilateral	Mammographic or palpable mass
Imaging findings	Spiculated mass	Spiculated mass or architectural distortion
Etiology	Unknown; may be associated with previous trauma, surgery, and breast implants.	Unknown
Histology	1. Poorly circumscribed mass *(Fig. 8.4.1)* 2. Locally infiltrative stromal neoplasm composed of long sweeping, intersecting fascicles of bland fibroblasts and myofibroblasts *(Fig. 8.4.2)* 3. Irregular "tongues" of lesion extend into fat *(Fig. 8.4.3)* 4. Hemorrhage around capillaries; no (or rare) mitotic figures *(Fig. 8.4.4)*	1. Bland spindle cells arranged in short, wavy, and storiform fascicles within collagenized and/or myxoid stroma *(Fig. 8.4.5)* 2. Generally more cellular than fibromatosis, but infiltrates around normal structures and into fat, similar to fibromatosis *(Fig. 8.4.6)* 3. Spindle cells have pale eosinophilic cytoplasm *(Fig. 8.4.7)* 4. Nuclei range from spindled to epithelioid with minimal atypia and rare mitoses *(Fig. 8.4.8)* 5. Mild mononuclear chronic inflammatory cells scattered within the stroma
Special studies	Cytoplasmic expression of actin and nuclear expression of β-catenin in 80% of cases. Desmin and S-100 expression may be detected in a minority of cells. Fibromatosis is negative for expression of cytokeratins, BCL-2, CD34, ER, PR, and AR.	Expresses nuclear p63 *(Fig. 8.4.9)* and p40 with variable intensity and distribution, some expression of cytokeratins, especially high molecular weight cytokeratins *(Fig. 8.4.10)*. Several antibodies against cytokeratins (including high molecular weight cytokeratins) usually required to establish the diagnosis. ER, PR, and HER2 negative.
Genetic abnormalities	May arise in patients with familial adenomatous polyposis coli, but most are sporadic. Activating mutations in β-catenin gene reported in 45% of cases, mutations in *FAP* or 5q loss reported in 33% of cases.	Recurrent mutations of *PIK3CA* and Wnt pathway genes

	Fibromatosis	Fibromatosis-like Metaplastic Carcinoma
Treatment	If anatomically feasible, wide local excision to obtain negative margins should be undertaken to minimize the risk of local recurrence. Radiation and chemotherapy ineffective and thus not indicated.	Excision to negative margins. Axillary lymph node sampling unnecessary unless a no special type carcinoma component is also present.
Clinical implication	Local recurrence in 20%–30% of cases, usually within 3 y of original diagnosis; lacks metastatic potential	Capable of local recurrence only

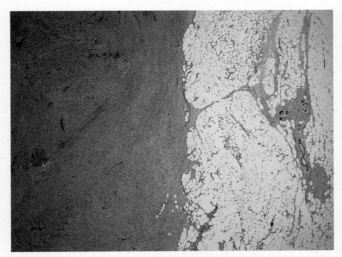

Figure 8.4.1 Fibromatosis having a nodular configuration yet an irregular interface with the surrounding fat.

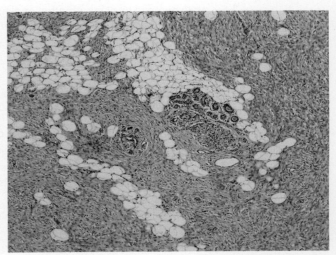

Figure 8.4.6 Fibromatosis-like metaplastic carcinoma is uniformly cellular, more so than is characteristic of fibromatosis.

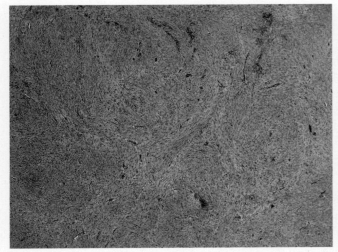

Figure 8.4.2 Intersecting fascicles of fibroblasts and myofibroblasts with myxoid stroma is characteristic of fibromatosis. Capillaries have a curvilinear arrangement and are associated with adjacent hemorrhage.

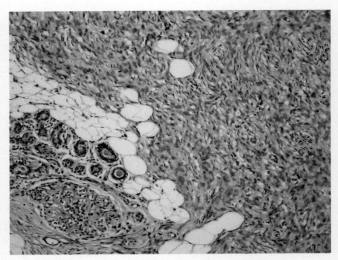

Figure 8.4.7 Plump nuclei of fibromatosis-like metaplastic carcinoma are more densely packed than the nuclei in fibromatosis.

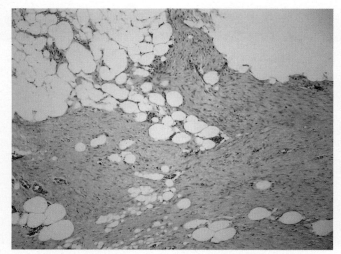

Figure 8.4.3 Fibromatosis has irregular "tongues" that extend into adjacent fat.

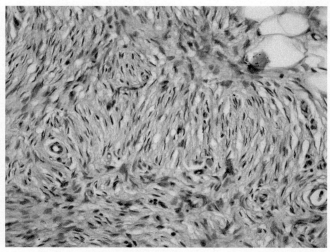

Figure 8.4.8 In addition to a spindle cell morphology, some of the nuclei of fibromatosis-like metaplastic carcinoma are distinctly epithelioid.

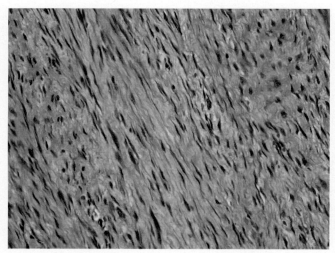

Figure 8.4.4 The nuclei of fibromatosis are elongated and wavy; note pericapillary hemorrhage.

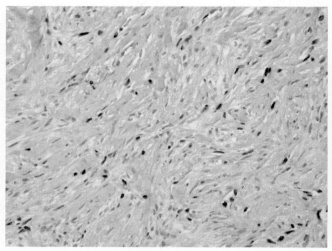

Figure 8.4.9 Nuclei of fibromatosis-like metaplastic carcinoma express p63.

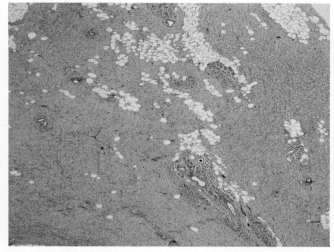

Figure 8.4.5 Fibromatosis-like metaplastic carcinoma infiltrates into fat and around normal lobular units.

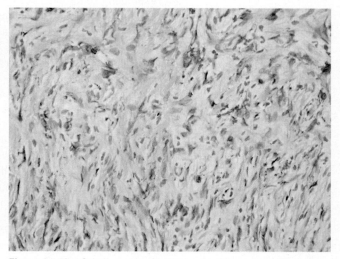

Figure 8.4.10 Spindled and epithelioid cells of fibromatosis-like metaplastic carcinoma express high molecular weight cytokeratin (CK5/6).

8 Stromal Lesions

	Myofibroblastoma	Fibromatosis
Age	Middle aged women, but wide age range (25–87 y); original description was in men	Wide age range, more common in females than males
Location	Anywhere in the breast, rarely multicentric, and bilateral	Most frequently arises from the pectoral fascia and extends into the breast but may occasionally originate within the breast parenchyma
Presentation	Solitary, slow-growing nodule, circumscribed and mobile, may be mistaken for fibroadenoma	Single, nontender, palpable mass; may be accompanied by skin retraction or dimpling; uncommonly bilateral
Imaging findings	Well-circumscribed homogeneously solid mass without associated microcalcifications	Often spiculated mass suspicious for carcinoma, but imaging may be normal
Etiology	Unknown	Association with previous trauma, surgery, and breast implants
Histology	1. Well-circumscribed nonencapsulated mass *(Fig. 8.5.1)* 2. Adipocytes may be an integral component or may define the edge of the lesion *(Fig. 8.5.2)* 3. Spindled to ovoid cells arranged in short, haphazard fascicles interspersed between thick bands of eosinophilic collagen *(Fig. 8.5.3)* 4. Wide morphologic spectrum may contain varying amounts of a benign adipocytic component resembling a spindle cell lipoma; appearance may be highly cellular *(Fig. 8.5.3)*, have epithelioid cells, myxoid change, or an extensive fibrous component resembling solitary fibrous tumor 5. Cells have abundant pale to eosinophic cytoplasm and round to oval nuclei *(Fig. 8.5.3)* 6. Necrosis absent and mitoses are rare *(Fig. 8.5.3)* 7. No entrapment of benign ducts or lobules *(Fig. 8.5.2)*	1. Usually a poorly circumscribed mass although occasionally a portion of the mass may be nodular *(Fig. 8.5.7)* 2. Locally infiltrative stromal neoplasm composed of long sweeping, intersecting fascicles of bland fibroblasts and myofibroblasts in variably edematous stroma *(Fig. 8.5.8)* 3. Variable cellularity, with the more cellular regions typically present at the periphery 4. Irregular tongues of fibroblasts extend into adjacent fat *(Figs. 8.5.8 and 8.5.9)* 5. May invade around normal structures 6. Lymphocytes often present at the infiltrative edge *(Fig. 8.5.10)* 7. Bland fibroblasts and myofibroblasts lack mitotic activity *(Fig. 8.5.11)*
Special studies	Diffuse expression of desmin, CD34, and/or smooth muscle actin *(Figs. 8.5.4–8.5.6)*. Variable expression of BCL-2, CD99, ER, PR, and AR, but negative for expression of keratin or p63.	Cytoplasmic expression of actin and nuclear expression of β-catenin in 80% of cases. Desmin and S-100 expression may be detected in a minority of cells. Fibromatosis is negative for expression of cytokeratins, BCL-2, CD34, ER, PR, and AR.

	Myofibroblastoma	**Fibromatosis**
Genetic abnormalities	Partial monosomy of 13q, monosomy 16q (same as spindle cell lipoma); deletion of 13q14 in most cases demonstrable by fluorescence in situ hybridization (FISH)	May arise in patients with *FAP*, but most are sporadic. Activating mutations in β-catenin gene reported in 45% of cases, mutations in *FAP* or 5q loss reported in 33% of cases.
Treatment	Complete excision unnecessary but may be performed for cosmesis	If anatomically feasible, wide local excision to obtain negative margins should be undertaken to minimize the risk of local recurrence. Radiation and chemotherapy ineffective and thus not indicated.
Clinical implication	No increased risk of breast cancer. No tendency for local recurrence.	Local recurrence in 20%–30% of cases, usually within 3 y of original diagnosis; lacks metastatic potential

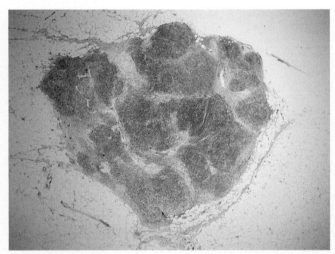

Figure 8.5.1   Myofibroblastoma consisting of a circumscribed proliferation of lobules of spindled cells intermixed with adipose tissue.

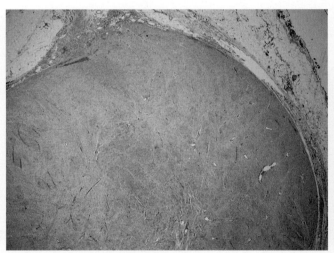

Figure 8.5.7   Fibromastosis showing a nodular architecture with dense collagen admixed with edematous stroma. Note a portion of the lesion is well-circumscribed.

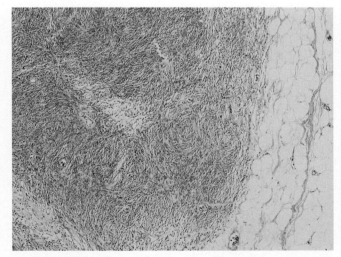

Figure 8.5.2   Spindled myofibroblasts are arranged in short intersecting fascicles with a sharp demarcation from adjacent fat.

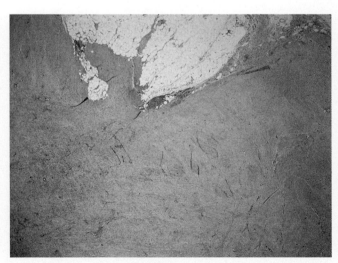

Figure 8.5.8   In other regions, irregular tongues of fibroblasts extend into adjacent fat; note the collections of lymphocytes at the periphery of lesion.

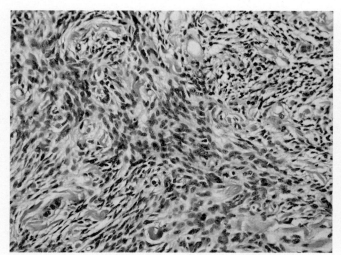

Figure 8.5.3   Nuclei of mofibroblastoma are often plump and arranged in short intersecting fascicles with intermixed dense collagen.

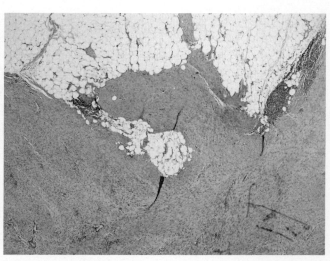

Figure 8.5.9   Keloidal type collagen is an integral component of fibromatosis. Irregular extension into fat and collections of lymphocytes at the periphery of the lesion are characteristic.

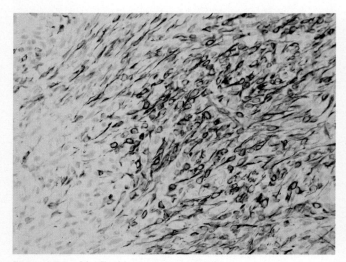

Figure 8.5.4   Myofibroblastoma expresses desmin.

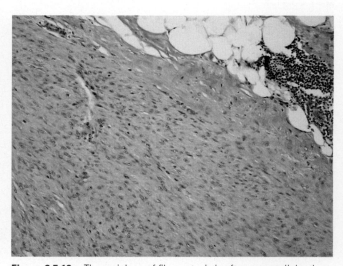

Figure 8.5.10   The periphery of fibromatosis is often more cellular than the central portion, consisting of bland spindle cells arranged in broad, sweeping fascicles.

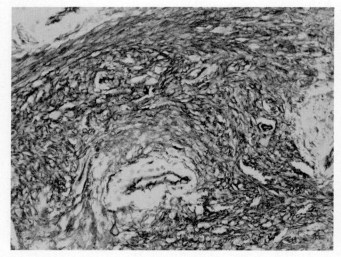

Figure 8.5.5   CD34 expression is characteristic of myofibroblastoma.

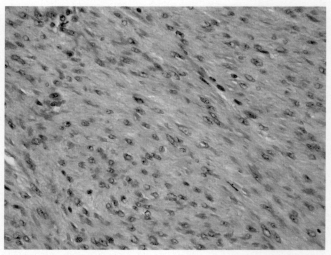

Figure 8.5.11   The nuclei of fibromatosis are bland, and mitotic activity is rare.

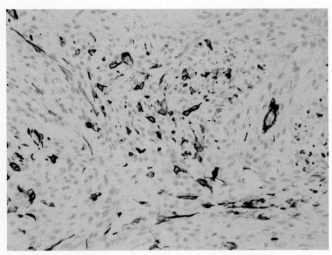

Figure 8.5.6   Smocth muscle actin is often expressed by myofibroblastoma.

	Epithelioid Myofibroblastoma	Pure Invasive Lobular Carcinoma
Age	Middle aged women, although wide age range (25–87 y), occasionally in men in association with gynecomastia	Middle age to older women averaging 57–65 y, slightly older than women with no special type carcinomas but incidence age overlaps with myofibroblastoma
Location	Anywhere in the breast, rarely multicentric, and bilateral	Anywhere in the breast; more commonly multicentric than other types of mammary carcinoma
Presentation	Solitary, slow-growing nodule, circumscribed and mobile, may be mistaken for fibroadenoma	Mammographic or less likely palpable abnormality
Imaging findings	Well-circumscribed homogeneously solid mass without associated microcalcifications	Spiculated mass or architectural distortion, calcifications infrequent, size frequently under-estimated by imaging studies
Etiology	Unknown	None, some studies suggest slight association with heavy alcohol consumption or hormone replacement therapy
Histology	1. Well-circumscribed nonencapsulated mass (Fig. 8.6.1) 2. Epithelioid cells simulating infiltrating lobular carcinoma interspersed between thick bands of eosinophilic collagen (Fig. 8.6.2) 3. Cells have abundant pale to eosinophic cytoplasm and round to ovoid nuclei with 1 or 2 small nucleoli (Fig. 8.6.3) 4. Necrosis absent, mitoses rare 5. No entrapment of benign ducts or lobules in the mass 6. Interface with the surrounding stroma is sharply circumscribed, but occasionally an irregular interface may be present with adipocytes often an integral component in these areas (Fig. 8.6.1)	1. Low combined histologic grade carcinoma composed of cells invading in a single-file arrangement or as single cells (Figs. 8.6.6 and 8.6.7) 2. Nuclei round to ovoid but may appear compressed by intracytoplasmic inclusions (Fig. 8.6.8) 3. Mitoses infrequent 4. May form a concentric pattern around normal structures (Fig. 8.6.6) 5. Associated tumor stroma is densely fibrotic (Fig. 8.6.6)
Special studies	Epithelioid cells of myofibroblastoma express ER (Fig. 8.6.4) but are negative for expression of cytokeratin (not shown). Desmin (Fig. 8.6.5), CD34, and BCL-2 are variably expressed as is smooth muscle actin.	Strongly expresses cytokeratin (Fig. 8.6.9); 80%–90% ER positive, HER2 negative
Genetic abnormalities	Partial monosomy of 13q, monosomy 16q (same as spindle cell lipoma); deletion of 13q14 in most cases demonstrable by FISH	Somatic truncating mutations within the E-cadherin gene (CDH1 at 16q22.1) combined with loss of heterozygosity and promotor methylation, gains on 1q and 16p; most frequently classified as luminal A by gene expression profiling
Treatment	These benign lesions do not require excision	Based on grade, stage, and receptor status

	Epithelioid Myofibroblastoma	**Pure Invasive Lobular Carcinoma**
Clinical implication	None	Favorable prognosis if pT1and pure (classic) low grade; distinctive metastatic pattern with spread to bone, gastrointestinal tract, uterus, ovary, serosal surfaces, and meninges

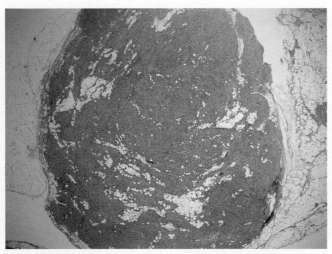

Figure 8.6.1   Myofibroblastoma is a sharply circumscribed benign proliferation of spindle cell and adipocytic components.

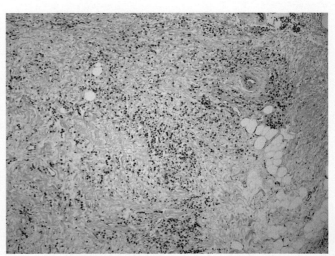

Figure 8.6.6   Invasive lobular carcinoma: Single cells infiltrate fibrous stroma and encircle normal structures.

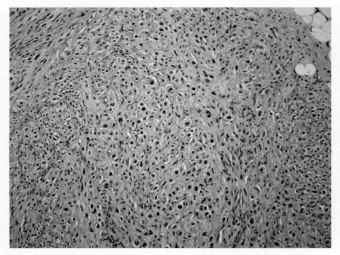

Figure 8.6.2   The proliferating cells of epithelioid myofibroblastoma show marked epithelioid characteristics simulating invasive lobular carcinoma.

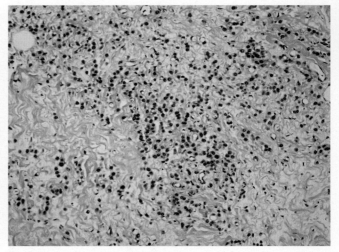

Figure 8.6.7   Invasive lobular carcinoma showing single file growth pattern and no spindle cell component.

8 Stromal Lesions

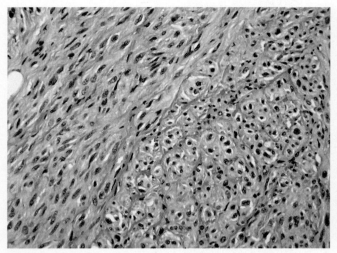

Figure 8.6.3   Epithelioid cells of myofibroblastoma, cut in cross section (right), and longitudinally (left). Invasive lobular carcinoma does not show the slightly spindled morphology of epithelioid myofibromblastoma (see Fig 8.6.8).

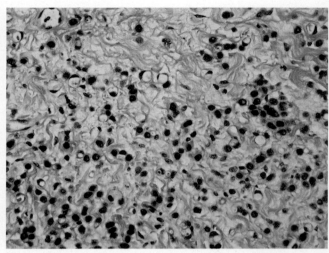

Figure 8.6.8   Intracytoplasmic inclusions are characteristic in invasive lobular carcinoma, compressing the nucleus.

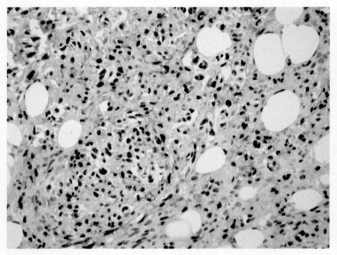

Figure 8.6.4   Epithelioid myofibroblastoma shows strong expression of ER, a potential pitfall in the distinction from invasive lobular carcinoma.

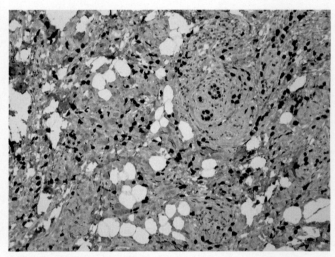

Figure 8.6.9   Invasive lobular carcinoma strongly expresses cytokeratin.

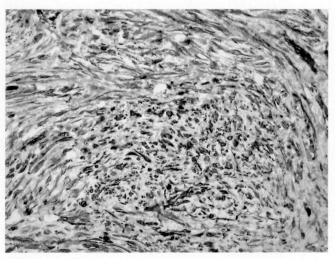

Figure 8.6.5   Strong desmin expression is characteristic of epithelioid myofibroblastoma.

	Myofibroblastoma	Fibromatosis-like Metaplastic Carcinoma
Age	Middle aged women, wide age range (25–87 y), occasionally in men in association with gynecomastia	Middle age women 50–70 y, age range overlaps with myofibroblastoma and invasive carcinomas of no special type
Location	Anywhere in the breast, rarely multicentric, and bilateral	Anywhere in the breast
Presentation	Solitary, slow-growing nodule, circumscribed and mobile, may be mistaken for fibroadenoma	Mammographic or palpable mass
Imaging findings	Well-circumscribed homogeneously solid mass without associated microcalcifications	Spiculated mass or architectural distortion
Etiology	Unknown	Unknown
Histology	1. Well-circumscribed nonencapsulated mass *(Fig. 8.7.1)* 2. Spindled to ovoid cells arranged in short, haphazard fascicles interspersed between thick bands of eosinophilic collagen *(Figs. 8.7.2 and 8.7.3)* 3. Wide morphologic spectrum may (a) contain varying amounts of a benign adipocytic component creating a spindle cell lipoma appearance, (b) be highly cellular, (c) have epithelioid cells, (d) an extensive fibrous component resembling solitary fibrous tumor, or (e) myxoid change 4. Cells have abundant pale to eosinophic cytoplasm and round to oval nuclei with 1 or 2 small nucleoli 5. Necrosis absent, mitoses rare 6. No entrapment of benign ducts or lobules within the mass 7. Interface with the surrounding stroma is usually sharply circumscribed *(Fig. 8.7.1)*, but occasionally an irregular interface may be present	1. Spindle cells arranged in short to long fascicles, may be arranged in a storiform pattern or interwoven *(Fig. 8.7.7)* 2. Neoplastic cells infiltrate around residual normal structures *(Fig. 8.7.8)* 3. Spindle cells have pale cytoplasm, and elongated, wavy nuclei with occasional epithelioid nuclei; nuclear atypia is minimal, and mitotic activity is rare *(Figs. 8.7.9 and 8.7.10)*
Special studies	Diffuse expression of desmin *(Fig. 8.7.4)* and CD34 *(Fig. 8.7.5)*. Usually expresses ER *(Fig. 8.7.6)* and variably expresses SMA, BCL-2, CD99, PR, and AR; negative for expression of cytokeratin.	Fibromatosis-like metaplastic carcinoma expresses cytokeratin *(Fig. 8.7.11)*, especially high molecular weight cytokeratins, and p63 *(Fig. 8.7.12)* as well as p40 with variable intensity and distribution. ER, PR, and HER2 negative. Use of a battery of cytokeratin antibodies may be required to establish the diagnosis.
Genetic abnormalities	Partial monosomy of 13q, monosomy 16q same as spindle cell lipoma; deletion of 13q14 in most cases demonstrable by FISH	Recurrent mutations of *PIK3CA* and Wnt pathway genes

	Myofibroblastoma	Fibromatosis-like Metaplastic Carcinoma
Treatment	Complete excision unnecessary but may be performed for cosmesis	Excision to negative margins. Axillary lymph node sampling unnecessary unless a component of no special type carcinoma is also present.
Clinical implication	No increased risk of breast cancer. No tendency for local recurrence.	Capable of local recurrence only

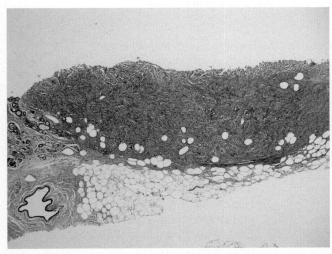

Figure 8.7.1   Myofibroblastoma showing a sharply circumscribed interface with adjacent fat and breast parenchyma.

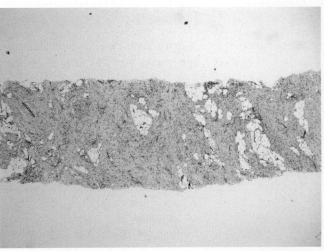

Figure 8.7.7   Paucicelluar spindle cell infiltrate of fibromatosis-like metaplastic carcinoma.

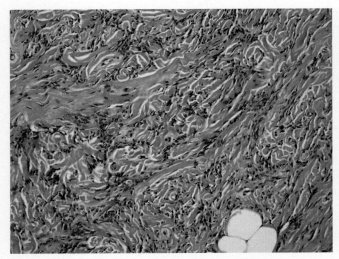

Figure 8.7.2   Short intersecting fascicles composed of bland spindle cells characterize myofibroblastoma.

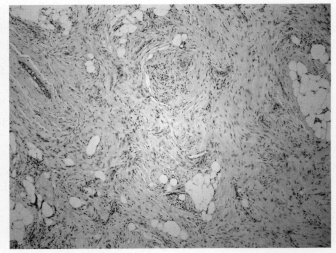

Figure 8.7.8   The spindle cells of fibromatosis-like metaplastic carcinoma infiltrate around preexisting ducts.

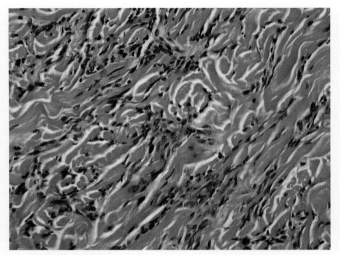

Figure 8.7.3   Bland spindled cells of myofibroblastoma intermixed with dense collagen.

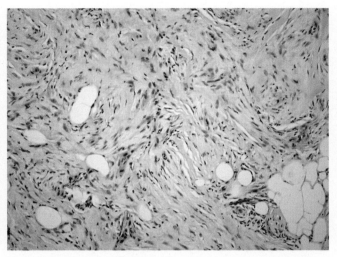

Figure 8.7.9   Neoplastic spindle cells are haphazardly arranged, and scattered stromal lymphocytes are common in fibromatosis-like metaplastic carcinoma.

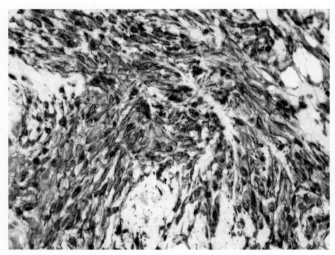

Figure 8.7.4   Desmin expression by myofibroblastoma.

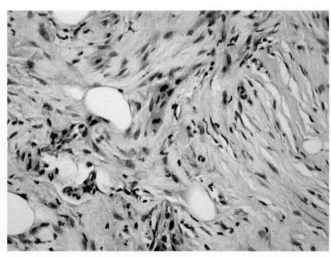

Figure 8.7.10   Fibromatosis-like metaplastic carcinoma cells have spindled, wavy nuclei with occasional epithelioid nuclei. Rare mitoses are present.

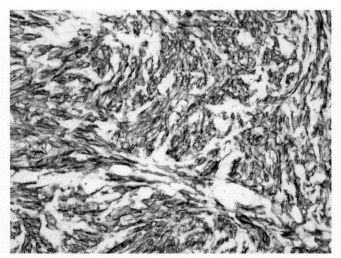

Figure 8.7.5   Myofibroblastoma characteristically expresses CD34.

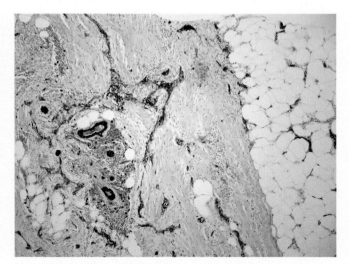

Figure 8.7.11   High molecular weight cytokeratin (detected using antibodies to CK903) is expressed by fibromatosis-like metaplastic carcinoma.

8 Stromal Lesions

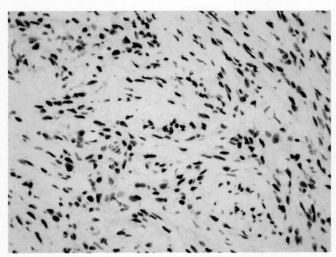

Figure 8.7.6   Estrogen receptor expression by myofibroblastoma should not be interpreted as evidence of an epithelial process.

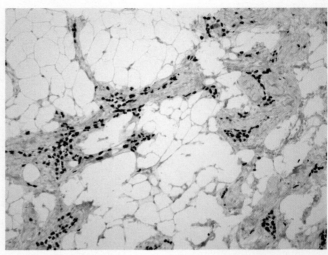

Figure 8.7.12   Diffuse expression of p63 is characteristic of fibromatosis-like metaplastic carcinoma.

	Post Biopsy Spindled Cell Nodule	Fibromatosis-like Metaplastic Carcinoma
Age	A woman of any age who has undergone a breast biopsy	Middle age women 50–70 y, overlapping age range for invasive carcinomas of no special type
Location	Anywhere in the breast	Anywhere in the breast
Presentation	Mass develops a few weeks after a sampling procedure	Mammographic or palpable mass
Imaging findings	Lobulated to spiculated mass	Spiculated mass or architectural distortion
Etiology	Local tissue response to recent fine needle aspiration, core needle biopsy procedure, or spontaneous infarction of an intraductal papilloma. Reported with greater frequency in patients with papillary and sclerosing lesions.	Unknown
Histology	1. Spindled cell proliferation often associated with fat necrosis *(Figs. 8.8.1 and 8.8.2)* 2. Spindle cells are present in edematous stroma and admixed with variable amounts of hemorrhage, hemosiderin, histiocytes, fat necrosis, and foreign body giant cells *(Figs. 8.8.3 and 8.8.4)* 3. Reactive atypia may be moderate *(Fig. 8.8.5)* 4. Usually well-circumscribed with a smooth interface between the spindle cell nodule and adjacent tissue	1. Spindle cell proliferation associated with dense, keloidal-type collagen with irregular extensions into adjacent tissue *(Fig. 8.8.6)* 2. Spindle cells are arranged in fascicles with an interwoven or storiform pattern, often entrapping normal structures *(Fig. 8.8.7)* 3. Mild nuclear atypia of wavy or epithelioid cells, rare mitotic figures present *(Fig. 8.8.8)*
Special studies	The proliferating cells in a reactive spindle cell nodule express muscle markers and vimentin but are negative for epithelial markers and p63.	Fibromatosis-like metaplastic carcinoma expresses cytokeratin *(Fig. 8.8.9)*, especially high molecular weight cytokeratins, and p63 *(Fig. 8.8.10)* as well as p40 with variable intensity and distribution. ER, PR, and HER2 negative. Use of a battery of cytokeratin antibodies may be required to establish the diagnosis.
Genetic abnormalities	None	Recurrent mutations of *PIK3CA* and Wnt pathway genes
Treatment	None required. Reactive spindle cell nodule regresses spontaneously.	Excision to negative margins. Axillary lymph node sampling unnecessary unless a component of no special type carcinoma is also present.
Clinical implication	None	Capable of local recurrence only

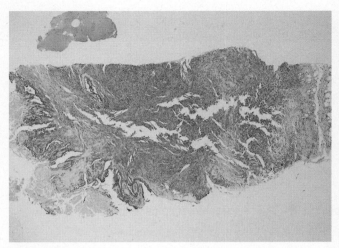

Figure 8.8.1   Spindle cell nodule, following biopsy of an intraductal papilloma: The central cellular area is associated with fat necrosis and residual fibrovascular fronds.

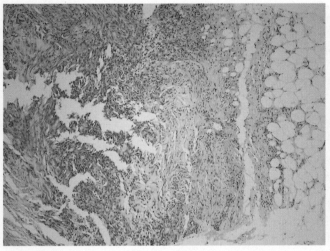

Figure 8.8.2   Exuberant granulation tissue-like appearance of a reactive spindle cell nodule, with adjacent fat necrosis.

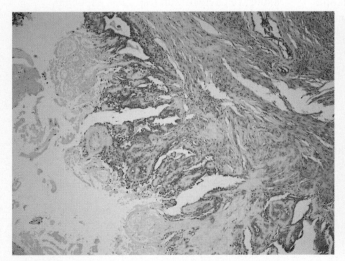

Figure 8.8.3   Proliferating spindle cells in an edematous stroma; note residual infarcted intraductal papilloma.

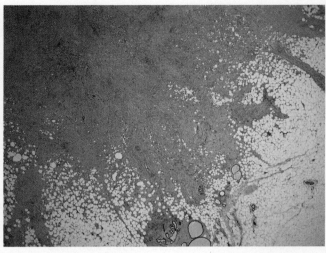

Figure 8.8.6   Fibromatosis-like metaplastic carcinoma: A dense collagenous nodule with extension into adjacent fat.

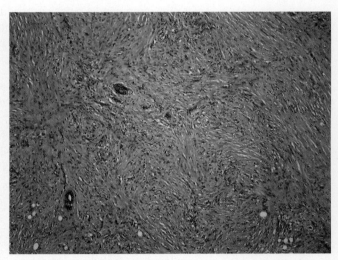

Figure 8.8.7   A proliferation of spindle cells entraps preexisting structures in fibromatosis-like metaplastic carcinoma.

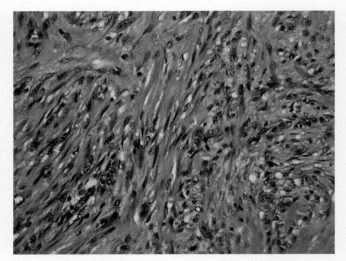

Figure 8.8.8   Nuclei vary from elongated and wavy to epithelioid; nuclear atypia is mild, and mitotic figures are rare in fibromatosis-like metaplastic carcinoma.

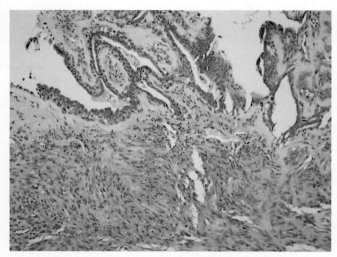

Figure 8.8.4   Edematous background, reactive spindled cells, and scattered lymphocytes adjacent to a previously biopsied intraductal papilloma.

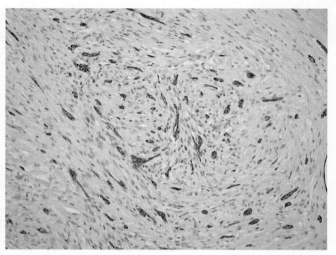

Figure 8.8.9   Fibromatosis-like metaplastic carcinoma expresses high molecular weight cytokeratin.

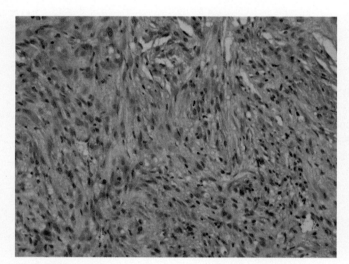

Figure 8.8.5   A cellular proliferation of spindle cells with mild reactive nuclear atypia associated with scattered lymphocytes characterizes a reactive spindle cell nodule secondary to a previous biopsy procedure.

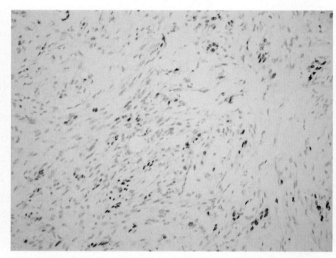

Figure 8.8.10   Expression of p63 is characteristic of fibromatosis-like metaplastic carcinoma.

8 Stromal Lesions

	Nonspecific Perilobular or Periductal Chronic Inflammation	Sclerosing Lymphocytic Lobulitis
Age	Any age	Middle aged women, although wide age range (25–87 y)
Location	Anywhere in the breast	Predominantly subareolar
Presentation	Incidental finding in a specimen removed for another indication; biproduct of a resolving inflammatory process (eg. mastitis, ruptured cyst)	Painless, palpable, ill-defined, or nodular breast mass that is predominantly subareolar; usually unilateral but may be bilateral and multifocal; has been described in male breasts
Imaging findings	Incidental finding, rarely architectural distortion	Usually palpable mass, frequently bilateral
Etiology	Unknown	Diabetes mellitus or other autoimmune disease, rarely precedes diagnosis of an autoimmune disorder
Histology	1. Concentric periductal and perilobular fibrosis *(Fig. 8.9.1)* 2. Maintains a regular distribution around mammary epithelial elements *(Fig. 8.9.2)* 3. Fibrosis consists of dense collagen, low cellularity *(Fig. 8.9.3)* 4. Lobular units may be atrophic 5. Intralobular connective tissue often edematous and contains lymphocytes *(Fig. 8.9.3)*	1. Dense fibrosis *(Fig. 8.9.4)* 2. Lymphocytic lobulitis and ductitis, predominantly composed of B cells which are polyclonal and may include follicles with germinal centers 3. Lymphocytic perivasculitis *(Fig. 8.9.4)* 4. Stromal "epithelioid fibroblasts" are a characteristic feature *(Figs. 8.9.5 and 8.9.6)*
Special studies	None	None
Genetic abnormalities	None	None
Treatment	None	None
Clinical implication	None	Also known as diabetic mastopathy and lymphocytic mastopathy, a distinctive clinico-pathologic entity strongly associated with autoimmune disease, likely representing an immune reaction to abnormal matrix production. Recurrences are common and can be ipsilateral, bilateral, or contralateral.

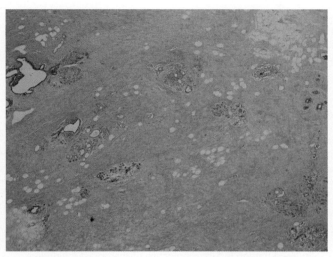

Figure 8.9.1 Nonspecific periductal and perilobular chronic inflammation are associated with dense stromal fibrosis. Mildly atrophic lobular units are evenly distributed in collagenous stroma.

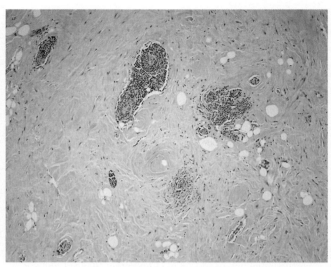

Figure 8.9.4 Markedly atrophic lobular units or "drop-out" of epithelial structures, and small vessels showing a dense surrounding lymphocytic infiltrate, are the hallmarks of sclerosing lymphocytic lobulitis.

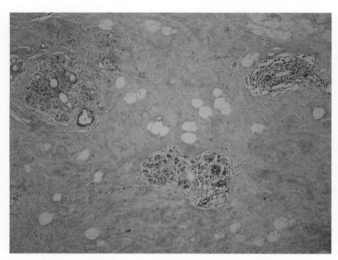

Figure 8.9.2 Lobular units showing mild atrophy and nonspecific lobular chronic inflammation.

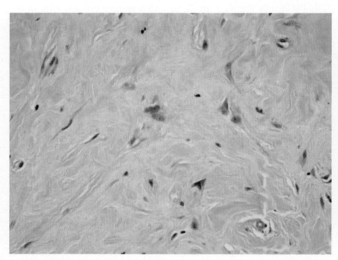

Figure 8.9.5 The stroma of sclerosing lymphocytic lobulitis contains dense collagen and epithelioid fibroblasts.

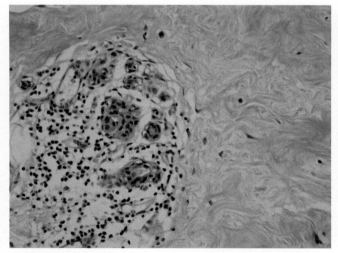

Figure 8.9.3 Connective tissue around lobular units is densely fibrotic, with only a few stromal cells. Scattered lymphocytes within an atrophic lobular unit.

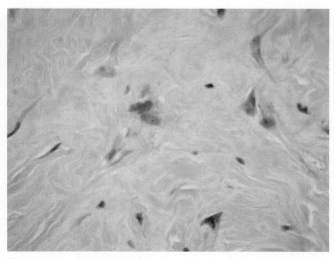

Figure 8.9.6 Epithelioid fibroblasts are the sine quo non of sclerosing lymphocytic lobulitis.

8 Stromal Lesions

SUGGESTED READINGS

Byrd BF Jr, Hartmann WH, Graham LS, et al. Mastopathy in insulin-dependent diabetics. *Ann Surg.* 1987;205:529–532.

Carlson JW, Fletcher CD. Immunohistochemistry for beta-catenin in the differential diagnosis of spindle cell lesions: analysis of a series and review of the literature. *Histopathology.* 2007;51:509–514.

Devouassoux-Shisheboran M, Schammel MD, Man YG, et al. Fibromatosis of the breast: age-correlated morphofunctional features of 33 cases. *Archiv Pathol Lab Med.* 2000;124:276–280.

Dubenko M, Breining D, Surks MI. Sclerosing lymphocytic lobulitis of the breast in a patient with Graves' disease. *Thyroid.* 2003;13:309–311.

Ely KA, Tse G, Simpson JF, et al. Diabetic mastopathy. A clinicopathologic review. *Am J Clin Pathol.* 2000;113:541–545.

Ferreira M, Albarracin CT, Resetkova E. Pseudoangiomatous stromal hyperplasia tumor: a clinical, radiologic and pathologic study of 26 cases. *Mod Pathol.* 2008;21:201–207.

Gobbi H, Tse G, Page DL, et al. Reactive spindle cell nodules of the breast after core biopsy or fine-needle aspiration. *Am J Clin Pathol.* 2000;113:288–294.

Lee KC, Chan JK, Ho LC. Histologic changes in the breast after fine-needle aspiration. *Am J Surg Pathol.* 1994;18:1039–1047.

Magro G, Michal M, Vasquez E, et al. Lipomatous myofibroblastoma: a potential diagnostic pitfall in the spectrum of the spindle cell lesions of the breast. *Virchows Arch.* 2000;437:540–544.

McMenamin ME, DeSchryver K, Fletcher CD. Fibrous lesions of the breast: A review. Int J Surg Pathol. 2000;8:99–108.

Nucci MR, Fletcher CDM. Myofibroblastoma of the breast: a distinctive benign stromal tumor. *Pathol Case Rev.* 1999;4:214–219.

Pauwels P, Sciot R, Croiset F, et al. Myofibroblastoma of the breast: genetic link with spindle cell lipoma. *J Pathol.* 2000;191:282–285.

Schwartz IS, Strauchen JA. Lymphocytic mastopathy. An autoimmune disease of the breast? *Am J Clin Pathol.* 1990;93:725–730.

Soler NG, Khardori R. Fibrous disease of the breast, thyroiditis, and cheiroarthropathy in type I diabetes mellitus. *Lancet.* 1984;1:193–195.

Tomaszewski JE, Brooks JS, Hicks D, et al. Diabetic mastopathy: a distinctive clinicopathologic entity. *Hum Pathol.* 1992;23:780–786.

Wargotz ES, Norris HJ, Austin RM, et al. Fibromatosis of the breast. A clinical and pathological study of 28 cases. *Am J Surg Pathol.* 1987;11:38–45.

9

Sentinel Lymph Nodes

	Benign Transport	Isolated Tumor Cells (ITC)
Age	Women of any age who undergo lymph node evaluation as part of breast cancer staging	Women of any age who undergo lymph node evaluation as part of breast cancer staging
Location	Subcapsular sinus of lymph node	Lymph node sinuses or parenchyma
Imaging findings	None or varying degrees of radionucleotide uptake identifying sentinel location	None or varying degrees of radionucleotide uptake identifying sentinel location
Etiology	Mechanical disruption and displacement secondary to prior breast biopsy	Lymphatic spread from mammary carcinoma
Histology	1. Single or small clusters of epithelial cells in subcapsular location *(Figs. 9.1.1 and 9.1.2)* 2. Pyknosis and prominent degenerative changes of the epithelium *(Fig. 9.1.3)* 3. Lack of stromal response 4. Hemosiderin, red blood cells (RBCs), histiocytes, cellular debris, and giant cells *(Fig. 9.1.3)* 5. Most often occurs following biopsy of papillary or micropapillary lesions; epithelial cell clusters in lymph node sinuses resemble previously biopsied lesion	1. Small clusters of epithelial cells present within the substance of lymph node and/or subcapsular sinus, usually with some associated stromal response *(Figs. 9.1.4 and 9.1.5)* 2. Solid nests or single cells, some with intracytoplasmic inclusions 3. Epithelial cells lack degenerative changes *(Fig. 9.1.5)* 4. Contiguous cells span a distance no larger than 0.2 mm and contain fewer than 200 tumor cells *(Fig. 9.1.6)* 5. Lack of associated hemosiderin-laden macrophages, RBCs, and giant cells
Special studies	None	None, but cytokeratin immunohistochemistry may be helpful when the tumor cells are widely dispersed
Treatment	Axillary lymph node dissection not indicated; treatment based on primary tumor characteristics	Axillary lymph node dissection not indicated; treatment based on primary tumor characteristics
Clinical implication	Lymph nodes that contain epithelial cell clusters resulting from benign transport are classified as pN0	Lymph node classified as pN0 (itc+)

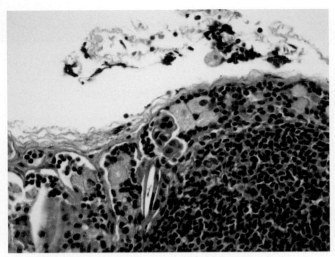

Figure 9.1.1   Benign transport of epithelium following a core needle biopsy procedure. The lymph node sinus contains degenerating epithelial cells, histiocytes, and cholesterol clefts.

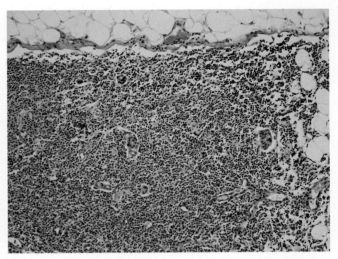

Figure 9.1.4   Isolated tumor cells; note scattered individual or small cellular clusters within the lymph node substance.

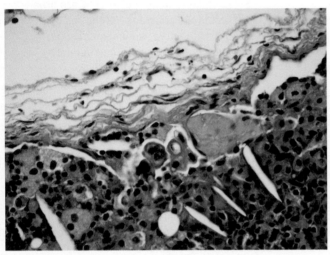

Figure 9.1.2   The degenerating epithelial cell clusters are associated with fragmented RBC's histiocytes and giant cells.

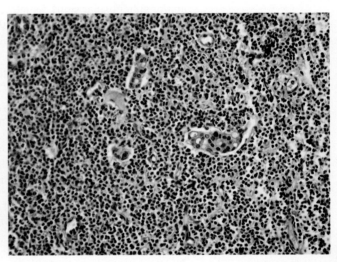

Figure 9.1.5   Isolated tumor cells present singly or in small clusters. Intracytoplasmic inclusions are evident.

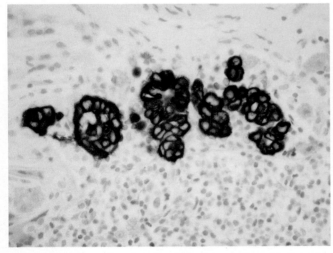

Figure 9.1.3   Expression of cytokeratin by degenerating epithelial cells; the presence of epithelial cells within the lymph node is the result of mechanical disruption and not metastasis. Evaluation of the local environment containing the cytokeratin positive cells allows proper diagnosis.

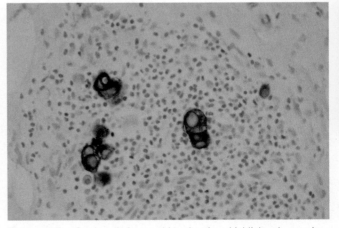

Figure 9.1.6   Cytokeratin immunohistochemistry highlights the paucity of tumor cells which number fewer than 200.

9 Sentinel Lymph Nodes

	ITC After Neoadjuvant Chemotherapy	Micrometastasis After Neoadjuvant Chemotherapy
Age	Women of any age who undergo lymph node evaluation as part of breast cancer staging	Women of any age who undergo lymph node evaluation as part of breast cancer staging
Location	Lymph node sinuses or parenchyma	Lymph node sinuses or parenchyma
Imaging findings	None or varying degrees of radionucleotide uptake identifying sentinel location	None or varying degrees of radionucleotide uptake identifying sentinel location
Etiology	Lymphatic spread from mammary carcinoma	Lymphatic spread from mammary carcinoma
Histology	1. Small clusters of epithelial cells present within the substance of a lymph node and/or subcapsular sinus, usually with some associated fibrosis and lymphoid depletion characteristic of neoadjuvant chemotherapy effect *(Fig. 9.2.1)* 2. Epithelial cells may show vacuolated cytoplasm *(Fig. 9.2.2)* 3. Cytokeratin immunohistochemistry shows scattered neoplastic cells, numbering fewer than 200 *(Fig. 9.2.3)*	1. Prominent sclerosis of lymph node with lymphoid depletion *(Fig. 9.2.4)* 2. Small clusters of epithelial cells are present within the substance of the residual nodal tissue and/or subcapsular sinus measuring more than 0.2 mm but not more than 2.0 mm *(Fig. 9.2.5)* 3. Stromal response within the residual lymph node is limited *(Fig. 9.2.5)*
Special studies	None, but cytokeratin may help with classification when the tumor cells are widely dispersed	None
Treatment	None, complete axillary dissection not indicated; additional treatment based on residual primary tumor characteristics	Complete axillary dissection not indicated if other sampled lymph nodes are negative for macrometastasis; treatment and prognosis are based on primary tumor characteristics
Clinical implication	Lymph node classified as ypN0 (itc+)	Classified as ypN1mi

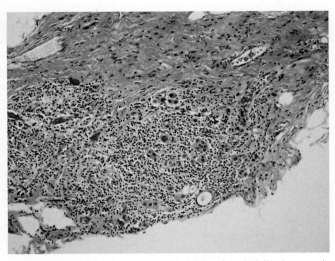

Figure 9.2.1 Isolated tumor cells within a lymph node following neoadjuvant chemotherapy.

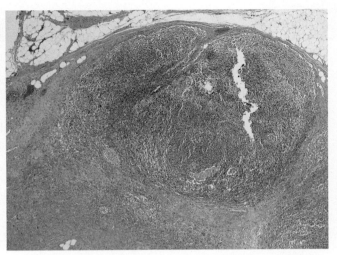

Figure 9.2.4 Micrometastasis following neoadjuvant chemotherapy: The lymph node shows characteristic dense fibrosis associated with chemotherapy effect.

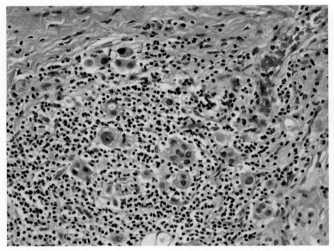

Figure 9.2.2 Scattered tumor cells number fewer than 200 and show cytoplasmic vacuolization, characteristic of treatment effect.

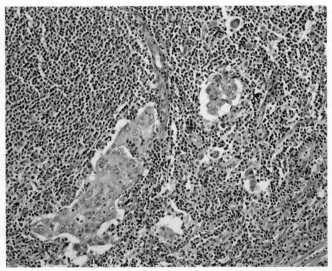

Figure 9.2.5 Neoplastic cell cluster measuring 2.2 mm, qualifying as a micrometastasis.

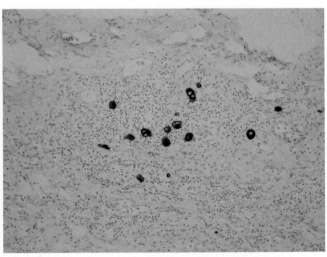

Figure 9.2.3 Cytokeratin immunohistochemistry highlights the paucicellular infiltrate in this lymph node.

9 Sentinel Lymph Nodes

	Micrometastasis	Macrometastasis
Age	Women of any age who undergo lymph node evaluation as part of breast cancer staging	Women of any age who undergo lymph node evaluation as part of breast cancer staging
Location	Lymph node sinuses or parenchyma	Lymph node sinuses or parenchyma
Imaging findings	None or varying degrees of radionucleotide uptake identifying sentinel location	None or varying degrees of radionucleotide uptake identifying sentinel location
Etiology	Lymphatic spread from mammary tumor	Lymphatic spread from mammary tumor
Histology	1. Small clusters of epithelial cells present within the substance of the lymph node and/or subcapsular sinus *(Fig. 9.3.1)* 2. Solid nests or single cells, some with intracytoplasmic inclusions *(Fig. 9.3.2)* 3. At least one focus of metastatic carcinoma or closely approximated clusters of carcinoma cells measuring more than 0.2 mm but not more than 2.0 mm, in nodal substance with or without involvement of subcapsular sinus, usually with some associated stromal response *(Fig. 9.3.3)*	1. Focus of metastatic carcinoma measuring more than 2.0 mm, present in nodal substance *(Fig. 9.3.4)* 2. Alteration of lymph node architecture *(Figs. 9.3.4–9.3.5)* 3. Usually associated with stromal response *(Fig. 9.3.5)*
Special studies	None routinely	None routinely. In borderline cases, hematoxylin and eosin (H&E) levels may help to establish presence of a more extensive lesion; accurate size determination (e.g., invasive lobular carcinoma) may be facilitated by cytokeratin immunohistochemistry
Treatment	Axillary node dissection not indicated if other sampled lymph nodes are negative for macrometastasis; treatment based on primary tumor characteristics	Complete axillary lymph node dissection frequently performed
Clinical implication	Classified as pN1mi	Single macrometastasis classified as pN1a; establishes propensity for distant metastasis

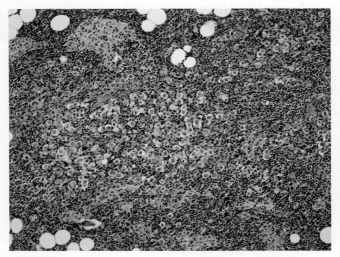

Figure 9.3.1 Micrometastasis consisting of a confluence of cells not larger than 2 mm.

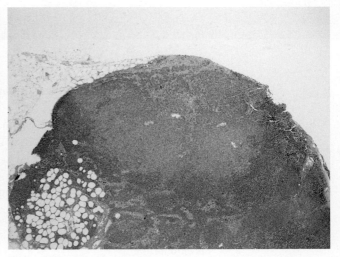

Figure 9.3.4 Macrometastasis, consisting of a solid nodule of tumor cells, measuring 4.0 mm.

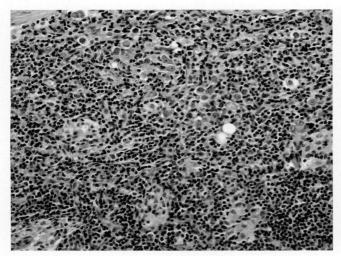

Figure 9.3.2 More than 200 tumor cells are present in this micrometastatic focus.

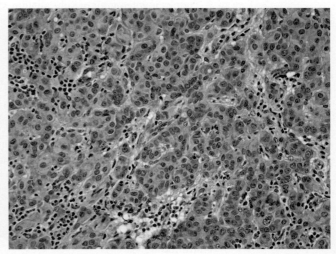

Figure 9.3.5 Confluent growth of a macrometastasis.

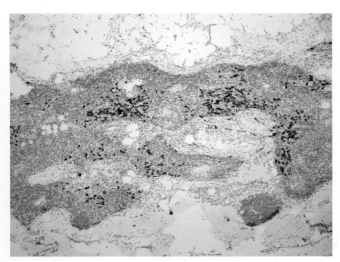

Figure 9.3.3 Cytokeratin immunohistochemistry shows several separate clusters of discontinuous metastatic tumor cells in this micrometastasis.

	Capsular Lymphatic Involvement by Carcinoma	Micrometastasis in Subcapsular Sinus
Age	Women of any age who undergo lymph node evaluation as part of breast cancer staging	Women of any age who undergo lymph node evaluation as part of breast cancer staging
Location	Lymphatic channel within lymph node capsule	Subcapsular sinus
Imaging findings	None or varying degrees of radionucleotide uptake identifying sentinel location	None or varying degrees of radionucleotide uptake identifying sentinel location
Etiology	Lymphatic spread from invasive mammary carcinoma	Lymphatic spread from invasive mammary carcinoma
Histology	1. A capsular lymphatic space containing carcinoma *(Figs. 9.4.1–9.4.3)* 2. Lacks involvement of subcapsular sinus or nodal substance	1. Metastatic carcinoma present immediately beneath the lymph node capsule in continuity with the lymphoid tissue *(Figs. 9.4.4 and 9.4.5)* 2. Focus of carcinoma measures more than 0.2 mm but not more than 2.0 mm; when amount is small and involves the fibrous capsule (e.g., ITC or micrometastasis), the differential diagnosis is intracapsular lymphatic involvement
Special studies	H&E levels may help to establish presence of carcinoma in lymph node proper in deeper sections. D2-40 immunohistochemistry may confirm intralymphatic location.	None required
Treatment	Axillary lymph node dissection not indicated; treatment based on primary tumor characteristics	If no larger than micrometastasis, axillary node dissection not indicated; treatment based on primary tumor characteristics
Clinical implication	Classified as pN0, although some studies suggest worse prognosis than pN0	Classified as pN1mi

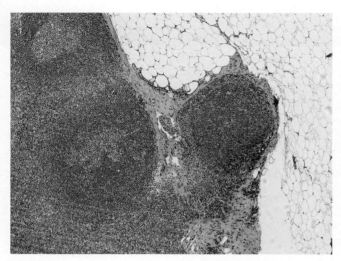

Figure 9.4.1   A lymphatic space within the capsule of the lymph node contains a cluster of neoplastic cells.

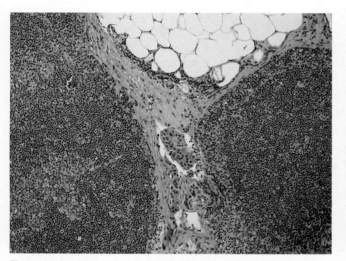

Figure 9.4.2   Note endothelial lining of lymphatic space. The presence of neoplastic cells in a capsular lymphatic space does not qualify as a metastasis (classified as pN0).

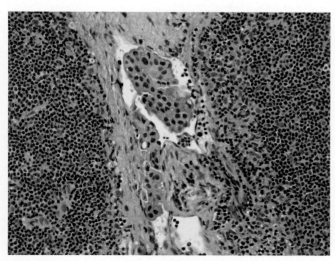

Figure 9.4.3   Tumor cluster within a lymphatic space. In this location, tumor cells are not considered ITC.

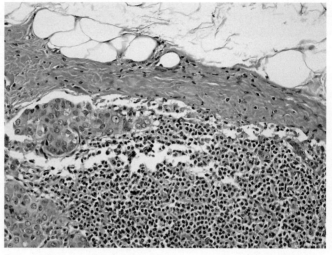

Figure 9.4.4   Micrometastasis, involving the subcapsular sinus and nodal parenchyma, and measuring 1.5 mm. Note tumor cells are beneath the lymph node capsule.

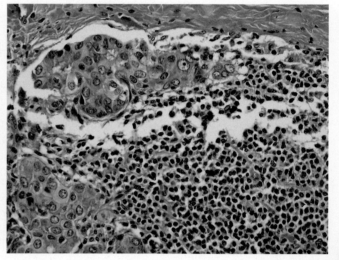

Figure 9.4.5   Micrometastasis, involving the subcapsular sinus and adjacent nodal parenchyma.

	Benign Glandular Inclusion	Micrometastasis
Age	Women of any age who undergo lymph node evaluation as part of breast cancer staging	Women of any age who undergo lymph node evaluation as part of breast cancer staging
Location	Lymph node capsule or nodal parenchyma	Lymph node sinuses or parenchyma
Imaging findings	None, usually incidental finding	None or varying degrees of radionucleotide uptake
Etiology	Most likely congenital origin; benign mammary epithelial elements in axillary lymph nodes and frequently in axillary tail of breast	Lymphatic spread from mammary carcinoma
Histology	1. Benign, round to ovoid glandular structures present in lymph node capsule and rarely in nodal substance *(Fig. 9.5.1)* 2. Two cell types are evident, an outer myo-epithelial layer with clear cytoplasm and an inner luminal cell layer *(Fig. 9.5.2)* 3. May demonstrate squamous metaplasia and contain keratin debris (not necrosis) *(Fig. 9.5.3)*	1. Focus of metastatic carcinoma measuring larger than 2.0 mm, present in nodal substance *(Fig. 9.5.5)* 2. Alteration of lymph node architecture and associated stromal response *(Figs. 9.5.5 and 9.5.6)*
Special studies	Immunohistochemical demonstration of two distinctive cell layers using antibodies to cytokeratin and markers of myoepithelial cells *(Fig. 9.5.4)*	None
Treatment	None	Axillary lymph node dissection not indicated; treatment based on primary tumor characteristics
Clinical implication	None	None; lymph node classified as pN1mi

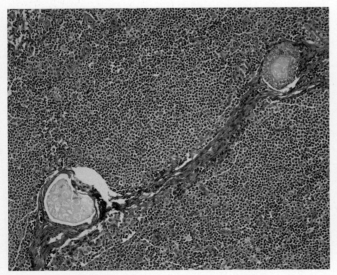

Figure 9.5.1 Benign glandular inclusion within lymph node septae. Eosinophilic material is keratin, not necrosis.

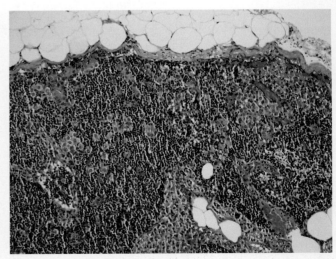

Figure 9.5.5 Neoplastic cells growing within nodal substance qualifying as micrometastasis based on size of 0.6 mm.

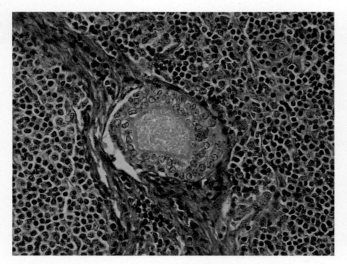

Figure 9.5.2   Two cell populations are evident in this benign glandular inclusion, a luminal epithelial layer and a basally located myoepithelial layer.

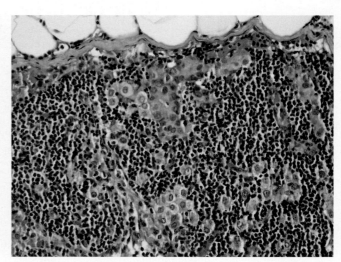

Figure 9.5.6   Micrometastasis consisting of clusters of carcinoma cells within the nodal substance.

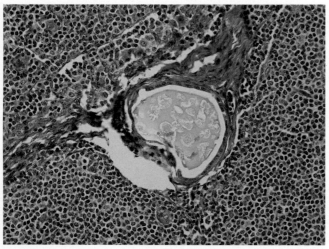

Figure 9.5.3   Benign glandular inclusion showing squamous metaplasia and associated keratin.

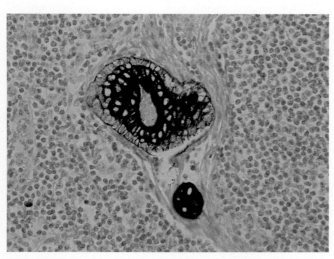

Figure 9.5.4   Cytokeratin immunohistochemistry highlights the luminal epithelium, while the myoepithelial cells are negative.

9 Sentinel Lymph Nodes

	Capsular Nevus	Capsular Lymphatic Involvement by Carcinoma
Age	Women of any age who undergo lymph node evaluation as part of staging for breast cancer	Women of any age who undergo lymph node evaluation as part of staging for breast cancer
Location	Within lymph node capsule	Lymphatic channel within lymph node capsule
Imaging findings	None	None or varying degrees of radionucleotide uptake identifying sentinel location
Etiology	Congenital presence of nevus cells within nodal capsule	Lymphatic spread from invasive mammary carcinoma
Histology	Small cluster of nevus cells within lymph node capsule *(Figs. 9.6.1 and 9.6.2)*	A capsular lymphatic space containing carcinoma without involvement of subcapsular sinus or nodal substance *(Figs. 9.6.4 and 9.6.5)*
Special studies	Immunohistochemical analysis shows lack of keratin expression and positivity for S-100 *(Fig. 9.6.3)*.	Deeper sections may help to establish the presence of carcinoma in lymph node proper. D2-40 immunohistochemistry may confirm intralymphatic location.
Treatment	None	Axillary lymph node dissection not indicated; treatment based on primary tumor characteristics
Clinical implication	None	Classified as pN0, although some studies suggest worse prognosis than pN0

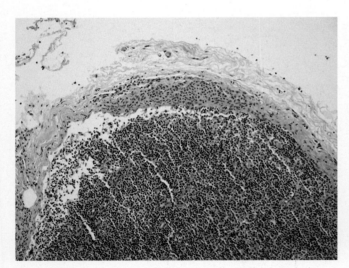

Figure 9.6.1 Capsular nevus: Bland nevus cells are tightly packed within the lymph node capsule.

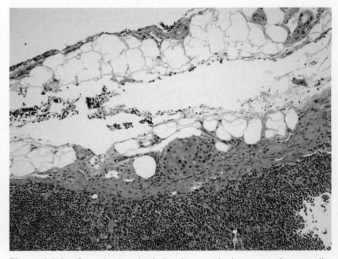

Figure 9.6.4 Capsular lymphatic involvement by breast carcinoma cells.

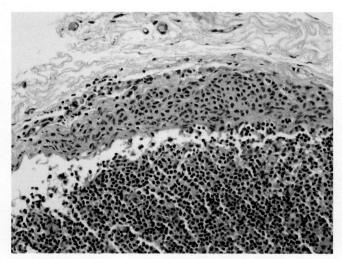

Figure 9.6.2   The nuclei of the nevus cells are slightly elongated, and there are no discrete cell borders.

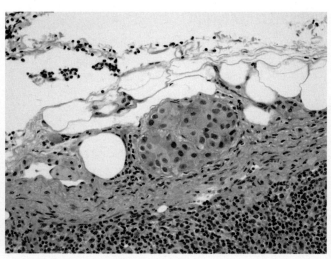

Figure 9.6.5   Capsular lymphatic involvement by breast carcinoma cells, showing distinct cell borders. This focus does not qualify as ITC.

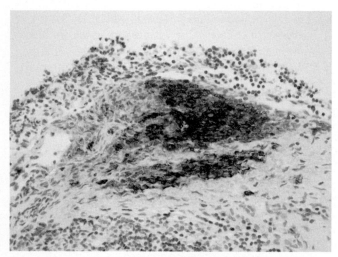

Figure 9.6.3   S-100 immunohistochemistry showing strong reactivity by the nevus cells; cytokeratin expression was absent (not shown).

SUGGESTED READINGS

Bleiweiss IJ, Nagi CS, Jaffer S. Axillary sentinel lymph nodes can be falsely positive due to iatrogenic displacement and transport of benign epithelial cells in patients with breast carcinoma. *J Clin Oncol.* 2006;24:2013–2018.

Carter BA, Jensen RA, Simpson JF, et al. Benign transport of breast epithelium into axillary lymph nodes after biopsy. *Am J Clin Pathol.* 2000;113:259–265.

Chagpar A, Middleton LP, Sahin AA, et al. Clinical outcome of patients with lymph node-negative breast carcinoma who have sentinel lymph node micrometastases detected by immunohistochemistry. *Cancer.* 2005;103:1581–1586.

Clare SE, Sener SF, Wilkens W, et al. Prognostic significance of occult lymph node metastases in node-negative breast cancer. *Ann Surg Oncol.* 1997;4:447–451.

Cronin-Fenton DP, Ries LA, Clegg LX, et al. Rising incidence rates of breast carcinoma with micrometastatic lymph node involvement. *J Natl Cancer Inst.* 2007;99:1044–1049.

Cserni G, Bianchi S, Vezzosi V, et al. The value of cytokeratin immunohistochemistry in the evaluation of axillary sentinel lymph nodes in patients with lobular breast carcinoma. *J Clin Pathol.* 2006;59:518–522.

de Mascarel I, MacGrogan G, Picot V, et al. Prognostic significance of immunohistochemically detected breast cancer node metastases in 218 patients. *Br J Cancer.* 2002;87:70–74.

Diaz NM, Vrcel V, Centeno BA, et al. Modes of benign mechanical transport of breast epithelial cells to axillary lymph nodes. *Adv Anat Pathol.* 2005;12:7–9.

Edge SB, Byrd, DR, Compton CC, et al., ed. *AJCC Cancer Staging Manual.* 7th ed. New York: Springer; 2010.

Fineberg S, Rosen PP. Cutaneous angiosarcoma and atypical vascular lesions of the skin and breast after radiation therapy for breast carcinoma. *Am J Clin Pathol.* 1994;102:757–763.

Fisher ER, Palekar A, Rockette H, et al. Pathologic findings from the National Surgical Adjuvant Breast Project (Protocol No. 4). V. Significance of axillary nodal micro- and macrometastases. *Cancer.* 1978;42:2032–2038.

Fisher ER, Swamidoss S, Lee CH, et al. Detection and significance of occult axillary node metastases in patients with invasive breast cancer. *Cancer.* 1978;42:2025–2031.

Giuliano AE, Dale PS, Turner RR, et al. Improved axillary staging of breast cancer with sentinel lymphadenectomy. *Ann Surg.* 1995;222:394–399; discussion 399–401.

Giuliano AE, Hawes D, Ballman KV, et al. Association of occult metastases in sentinel lymph nodes and bone marrow with survival among women with early-stage invasive breast cancer. *JAMA.* 2011;306:385–393.

Gobardhan PD, Elias SG, Madsen EV, et al. Prognostic value of micrometastases in sentinel lymph nodes of patients with breast carcinoma: a cohort study. *Ann Oncol.* 2009;20:41–48.

Huvos AG, Hutter RV, Berg JW. Significance of axillary macrometastases and micrometastases in mammary cancer. *Ann Surg.* 1971;173:44–46.

Kaufmann M, Morrow M, von Minckwitz G, et al. Locoregional treatment of primary breast cancer: consensus recommendations from an International Expert Panel. *Cancer.* 2010;116:1184–1191.

Layfield LJ, Mooney E. Heterotopic Epithelium in an Intramammary Lymph Node. *Breast J.* 2000;6:63–67.

Lyman GH, Giuliano AE, Somerfield MR, et al. American Society of Clinical Oncology guideline recommendations for sentinel lymph node biopsy in early-stage breast cancer. *J Clin Oncol.* 2005;23:7703–7720.

National Comprehensive Cancer Network (NCCN). NCCN guidelines. In: *Journal of the National Comprehensive Cancer Network.* Cold Spring Harbor, NY: Harborside Press; 2011.

Pickren JW. Significance of occult metastases. A study of breast cancer. *Cancer.* 1961;14:1266–1271.

Pugliese MS, Beatty JD, Tickman RJ, et al. Impact and outcomes of routine microstaging of sentinel lymph nodes in breast cancer: significance of the pN0(i+) and pN1mi categories. *Ann Surg Oncol.* 2009;16:113–120.

Rosen PP, Saigo PE, Braun DW Jr, et al. Occult axillary lymph node metastases from breast cancers with intramammary lymphatic tumor emboli. *Am J Surg Pathol.* 1982;6:639–641.

Turner RR, Weaver DL, Cserni G, et al. Nodal stage classification for breast carcinoma: improving interobserver reproducibility through standardized histologic criteria and image-based training. *J Clin Oncol.* 2008;26:258–263.

Weinberg ES, Dickson D, White L, et al. Cytokeratin staining for intraoperative evaluation of sentinel lymph nodes in patients with invasive lobular carcinoma. *Am J Surg.* 2004;188:419–422.

Wilkinson EJ, Hause LL, Hoffman RG, et al. Occult axillary lymph node metastases in invasive breast carcinoma: characteristics of the primary tumor and significance of the metastases. *Pathol Annu.* 1982;17(Pt 2):67–91.

10

Vascular Lesions

	Perilobular Capillary Hemangioma	Angiolipoma
Age	Middle age or older women	Any age
Location	Anywhere in the breast	Breast subcutaneous tissue, rarely mammary parenchyma
Presentation	Incidental finding	Painful dermal nodules, may be multiple
Imaging findings	None or small nodular density	None or rarely nodular density
Etiology	Unknown	Unknown
Histology	1. Well-circumscribed proliferation of thin-walled capillaries that may involve the intralobular or extralobular stroma *(Fig. 10.1.1)* 2. Incorporates lobular unit(s) but does not invade epithelial structures *(Figs. 10.1.2–10.1.4)* 3. Capillaries are lined by attenuated endothelial cells with small nuclei devoid of atypia *(Fig. 10.1.5)*	1. Well-circumscribed lesion composed of an admixture of mature adipose tissue and noninfiltrative small vascular spaces *(Figs. 10.1.6 and 10.1.7)* 2. Vascular spaces may be compressed and slit-like *(Fig. 10.1.8)* 3. Adipose tissue is an integral component of the lesion *(Fig. 10.1.9)* 4. Vascular spaces lined by bland endothelial cells containing intravascular hyaline microthrombi *(Fig. 10.1.10)*
Special studies	None	None
Treatment	None, excision unnecessary	None, excision not required unless painful
Clinical implication	None, benign incidental finding	None

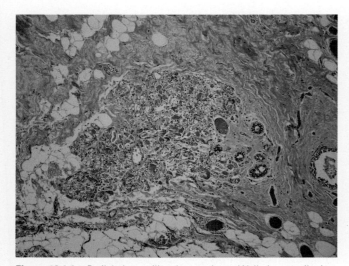

Figure 10.1.1 Perilobular capillary hemangioma: Well-circumscribed proliferation of small vessels that incorporates a lobular unit.

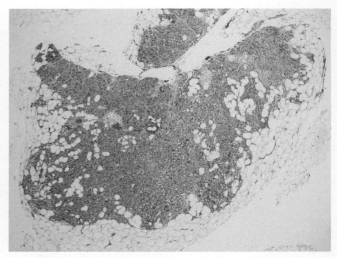

Figure 10.1.6 Angiolipoma is nodular and well-circumscribed, composed of mature adipose tissue and noninfiltrative, small vessels.

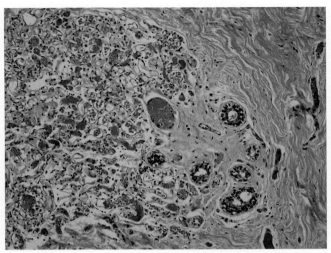

Figure 10.1.2   The capillaries may involve intralobular and extralobular stroma in a perilobular capillary hemangioma.

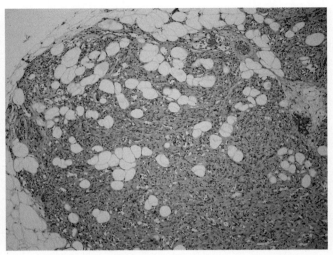

Figure 10.1.7   In angiolipoma, the vessels are small, densely packed, and congested.

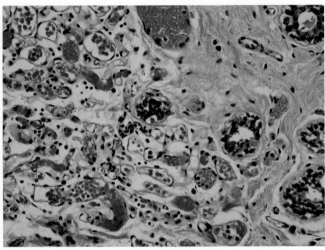

Figure 10.1.3   The thin-walled capillaries of perilobular capillary hemangioma incorporate the lobular unit(s) but do not invade epithelial structures.

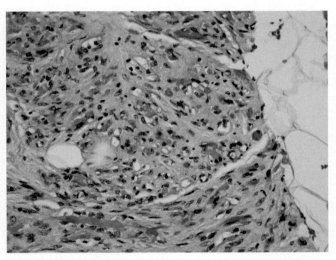

Figure 10.1.8   The small vascular spaces in angiolipoma are tightly opposed resembling granulation tissue.

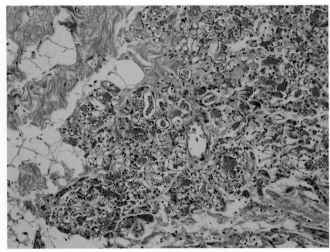

Figure 10.1.4   Perilobular capillary hemangioma has a lobulated interface with the surrounding mammary parenchyma and remains circumscribed in areas involving extralobular stroma.

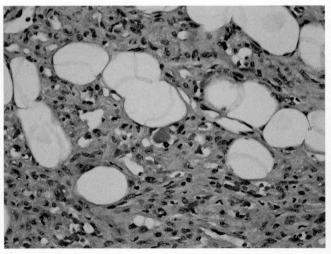

Figure 10.1.9   Bland endothelial cells line the vessels of angiolipoma; microthrombi are common.

10 Vascular Lesions

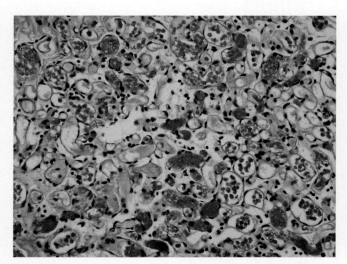

Figure 10.1.5   The capillaries of perilobular capillary hemangioma are lined by attenuated endothelial cells with small nuclei devoid of atypia.

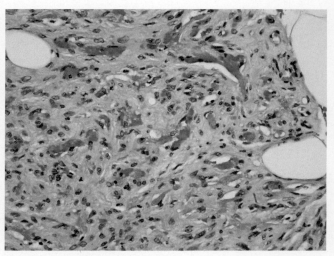

Figure 10.1.10   The endothelial cells are occasionally spindled in angiolipoma.

	Perilobular Capillary Hemangioma	Atypical Vascular Lesion
Age	Middle age or older women	Middle age and older women, (usually sixth decade)
Location	Anywhere in the breast	Breast skin
Presentation	Incidental finding	Papules or plaques appearing several years (average 3–4 y) following radiation therapy; red-brown or pink
Imaging findings	None, rarely nodular density	May show skin thickening
Etiology	Unknown	Radiation exposure, often for breast cancer
Histology	1. Well-circumscribed proliferation of thin-walled capillaries that may involve the intralobular or extralobular stroma *(Figs. 10.2.1–10.2.3)* 2. Incorporate lobular unit(s) but do not invade epithelial structures *(Figs. 10.2.1–10.2.4)* 3. Capillaries are lined by attenuated endothelial cells with small nuclei devoid of atypia *(Fig. 10.2.5)*	1. Localized, often wedge-shaped collection of haphazardly arranged and focally dilated vascular spaces in dermis. May be very subtle *(Figs. 10.2.6 and 10.2.7)* 2. Vascular spaces may have a complex branching pattern and may be anastomosing *(Fig. 10.2.8)* 3. The vascular spaces are confined to the dermis and lined by single layer of plump endothelial cells with nuclear hobnailing and hyperchromasia, but no mitoses *(Fig. 10.2.9)* 4. Vessels suggest an infiltrative process; however, overall small size and circumscription support a diagnosis of atypical vascular lesion *(Fig. 10.2.7)*
Special studies	None	None to distinguish from capillary hemangioma
Treatment	None, excision unnecessary	Atypical vascular lesions should be excised with the aim of obtaining negative margins
Clinical implication	None, benign incidental finding	Following complete excision, the majority pursue a benign clinical course with a few cases reportedly recurring locally or progressing to angiosarcoma

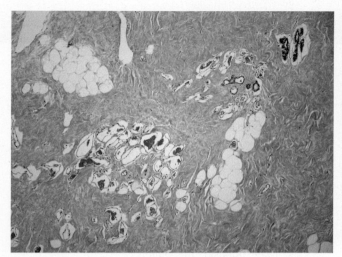

Figure 10.2.1   This perilobular capillary hemangioma is an inconspicuous proliferation of dilated capillaries present in the specialized and adjacent nonspecialized connective tissue of several adjacent lobular units.

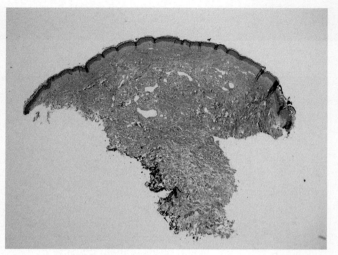

Figure 10.2.6   Atypical vascular lesion, showing a characteristic wedge-shaped collection of haphazardly arranged and focally dilated vascular spaces in the dermis.

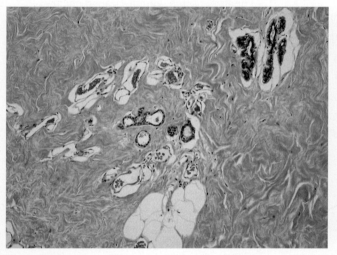

Figure 10.2.2   The capillaries may involve intralobular and extralobular stroma, but the lesion is architecturally circumscribed.

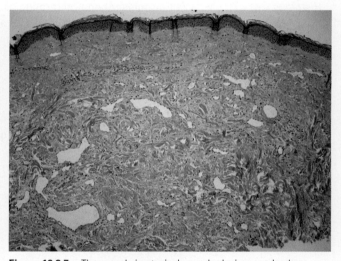

Figure 10.2.7   The vessels in atypical vascular lesions are haphazardly arranged and do not contain red blood cells: there is no red cell extravasation.

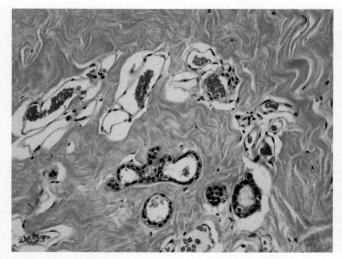

Figure 10.2.3   The thin-walled capillaries of perilobular capillary hemangioma frequently incorporate the acini of lobular units but do not invade epithelial structures.

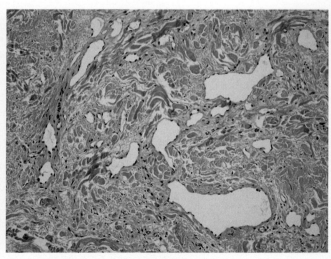

Figure 10.2.8   The vascular spaces are irregularly placed and separated by small bundles of dermal collagen.

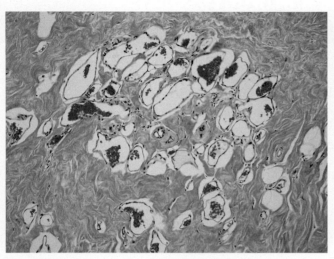

Figure 10.2.4 Attenuated endothelial cells with small nuclei devoid of atypia line the capillaries of perilobular capillary hemangioma.

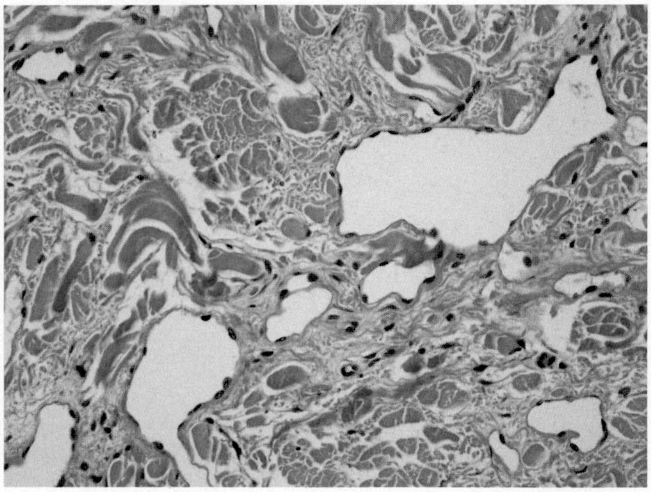

Figure 10.2.9 An atypical vascular lesion lined by plump endothelial cells. Nuclear hobnailing and hyperchromasia are frequently observed; however, overt nuclear atypia, endothelial multilayering, mitotic activity, and infiltration of the subcutis and breast parenchymal structures are absent.

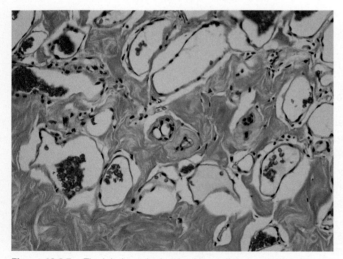

Figure 10.2.5 The lobular units involved by perilobular capillary hemangioma are frequently atrophic.

	Atypical Vascular Lesion	Postradiation Angiosarcoma, Low-Grade Histology
Age	Middle age and older women (usually sixth decade)	Women over 50 y of age (approximately 20 y older than women with primary angiosarcoma), time to diagnosis ranges from 2.5 to 11.5 y (median 4.5 y) after radiation therapy; risk of developing postradiation angiosaroma is approximately 0.3%
Location	Breast skin	Breast skin, may extend into adjacent mammary parenchyma
Presentation	Papules or plaques appearing several years (average 3–4 y) following radiation therapy; red-brown or pink	Multifocal, cutaneous, purple-blue and erythematous plaques, papules, or nodules within the radiation field which may secondarily involve adjacent breast parenchyma
Imaging findings	Skin thickening; none	None or skin thickening; associated ill-defined density with involvement of breast parenchyma; magnetic resonance imaging (MRI) may be useful in defining the size
Etiology	Radiation exposure, usually for breast cancer	Radiation treatment for breast cancer
Histology	1. Localized, often wedge-shaped collection of haphazardly arranged and focally dilated vascular spaces in dermis. May be very subtle (Fig. 10.3.1) 2. Vascular spaces may have a complex branching pattern and be anastomosing (Figs. 10.3.2 and 10.3.3) 3. The vascular spaces are confined to the dermis and lined by a single layer of plump endothelial cells with nuclear hobnailing and hyperchromasia, but no mitoses (Fig. 10.3.4) 4. Vascular spaces separated by small bundles of dermal collagen 5. Vessels suggest an infiltrative process; however, overall small size and circumscription support a diagnosis of atypical vascular lesion	1. Complex, anastomosing vascular channels that infiltrate the dermis and/or the breast parenchyma (Figs. 10.3.5 and 10.3.6) 2. Well-defined vascular spaces lined by cells with prominent nuclei that protrude into the vascular lumen (Figs. 10.3.7 and 10.3.8) 3. Subtle permeation of adipose tissue mimics angiolipoma 4. May contain atypical vascular lesion-like areas in the periphery of the lesion; distinction from atypical vascular lesion on core biopsy specimen may be difficult, requiring excision for diagnosis
Special studies	Absent c-myc expression by immunohistochemistry and lack of myc amplification by fluorescence in situ hybridization (FISH) distinguish from angiosarcoma with high specificity; immunohistochemistry for ERG may reassure a limited extent of the process and circumscription but does not distinguish from angiosarcoma. Immunohistochemical staining for vascular markers does not distinguish from angiosarcoma.	MYC amplification present in >50% of postradiation angiosarcomas but absent in atypical vascular lesions. Immunohistochemistry for c-myc shows nearly 100% concordance with MYC amplification as detected by FISH. Immunohistochemical expression of vascular markers does not distinguish from atypical vascular lesions.

	Atypical Vascular Lesion	**Postradiation Angiosarcoma, Low-Grade Histology**
Treatment	Atypical vascular lesions should be excised with the aim of obtaining negative margins. When diagnosed on needle core biopsy, excision is generally warranted to exclude angiosarcoma.	Total mastectomy; wide excision alone is associated with high recurrence rates. Radiotherapy and chemotherapy ineffective.
Clinical implication	Following complete excision, the majority pursue a benign clinical course with a few cases reportedly recurring locally or progressing to angiosarcoma. Distinction from angiosarcoma is critical to avoid excessive surgery and inappropriate prognostication.	Postradiation angiosarcoma, regardless of grade, has a poor prognosis with a mean survival of 1–2 y

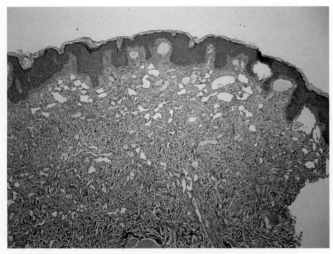

Figure 10.3.1 Atypical vascular lesion, showing numerous variably sized, haphazardly arranged vascular spaces the in dermis.

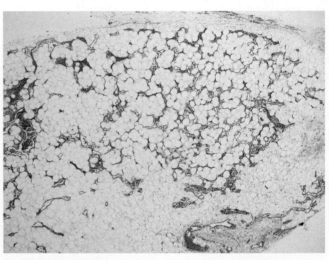

Figure 10.3.5 Haphazardly arranged anastomosing vascular channels infiltrate fat in postradiation angiosarcoma with low-grade histology.

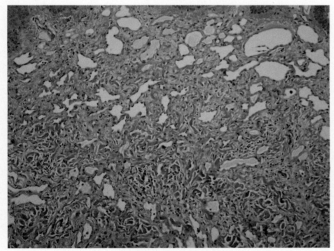

Figure 10.3.2 The vessels in atypical vascular lesions are irregularly placed and variably shaped but do not contain red blood cells. There is no red cell extravasation in the intervening stroma.

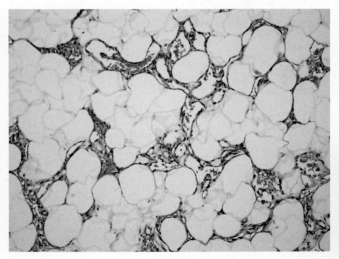

Figure 10.3.6 Dilated anastomosing vascular spaces contain erythrocytes in low-grade angiosarcoma.

10 Vascular Lesions

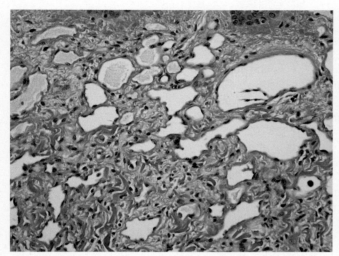

Figure 10.3.3   In atypical vascular lesions, plump endothelial cells line the vascular spaces and nuclear hobnailing and hyperchromasia are frequently present; however, overt nuclear atypia, endothelial multilayering, mitotic activity, and infiltration of the subcutis and breast parenchymal structures are absent.

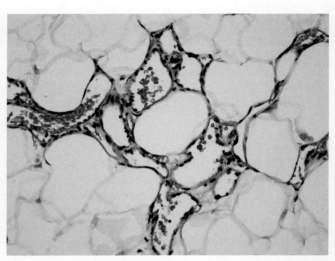

Figure 10.3.7   Low-grade angiosarcoma: Vasoformative spaces are lined by plump endothelial cells that have hyperchromatic nuclei that bulge into the lumen.

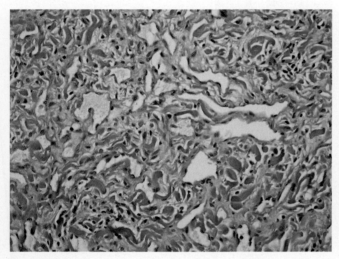

Figure 10.3.4   Scattered small bundles of dermal collagen are present between the irregularly placed vascular spaces.

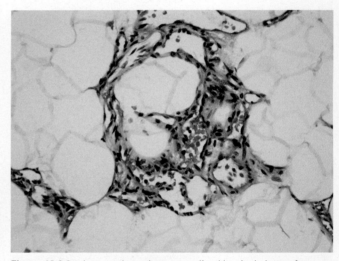

Figure 10.3.8   Low-grade angiosarcoma, lined by single layer of enlarged endothelial cells, without tufting or mitotic activity.

	Primary Angiosarcoma	Postradiation Angiosarcoma
Age	Women age 17–70 y (median, 38 y).	Women over 50 y of age (approximately 20 y older than women with primary angiosarcoma), time to diagnosis ranges from 2.5 to 11.5 y (median 4.5 y) after radiation therapy; risk of developing postradiation angiosaroma is approximately 0.3%
Location	Breast or skin of breast	Breast skin, may extend into adjacent mammary parenchyma
Presentation	Solitary, painless mass (often >5 cm); deep location may have no external signs or symptoms	Multifocal, cutaneous, purple-blue and erythematous plaques, papules, or nodules within the field of radiation which may secondarily involve adjacent breast parenchyma
Imaging findings	Architectural distortion without microcalcifications or a large ill-defined density within the breast parenchyma. MRI may be useful in defining the size.	None or skin thickening; associated ill-defined density with involvement of breast parenchyma; MRI may be useful in defining the size
Etiology	Unknown, sporadic	Radiation treatment for breast cancer
Histology	1. Histologic appearance ranges from well-differentiated, obviously vasoformative lesions to solid, poorly differentiated neoplasms. Full histologic spectrum may be seen in individual lesions *(Figs. 10.4.1–10.4.8)* 2. Well-differentiated areas show complex, anastomosing vascular channels that infiltrate the dermis and/or the breast parenchyma *(Figs. 10.4.1 and 10.4.2)*	1. Histologic appearance ranges from well-differentiated, obviously vasoformative lesions to solid, poorly differentiated neoplasms. Full histologic spectrum may be seen in individual lesions; however, most postradiation angiosarcomas are predominantly high grade *(Figs. 10.4.5–10.4.9)* 2. Well-differentiated areas show complex, anastomosing vascular channels that infiltrate the dermis and/or the breast parenchyma; Vascular spaces are well-defined and lined by cells with prominent nuclei that protrude into the vascular lumen; endothelial tufting is minimal and papillary formations are absent; may subtly permeate adipose tissue simulating angiolipoma

	Primary Angiosarcoma	Postradiation Angiosarcoma
	3. Vascular spaces are well-defined and lined by cells with prominent nuclei that protrude into the vascular lumen *(Figs. 10.4.3 and 10.4.4)* 4. Endothelial tufting is minimal and papillary formations are absent *(Figs. 10.4.4 and 10.4.5)* 5. May subtly permeate adipose tissue simulating angiolipoma *(Fig. 10.4.2)* 6. Less-differentiated variants, whether primary or in the postradiation setting, show prominent endothelial cell tufting, papillary formations, or multilayered growth of obviously malignant, mitotically active cells 7. Solid or spindle cell foci, blood lakes, necrosis, and limited evidence of vascular differentiation are characteristic of poorly differentiated tumors in both the primary and postradiation setting	3. Less-differentiated variants show prominent endothelial cell tufting, papillary formations, or multilayered growth of obviously malignant, mitotically active cells *(Figs. 10.4.7–10.4.9)* 4. Solid or spindle cell foci, blood lakes, and necrosis are characteristic of poorly differentiated tumors, and some may show limited evidence of vascular differentiation 5. Variable numbers of slit-like spaces containing intraluminal or extravasated erythrocytes or interstitial hemorrhage with the formation of blood lakes are typically, but not always, present in poorly differentiated lesions *(Figs. 10.4.8 and 10.4.9)* 6. Extravasated red blood cells are prominent *(Fig. 10.4.8)*
Special studies	MYC amplification less frequently present than in radiation-induced angiosarcomas. Immunohistochemistry for c-myc shows nearly 100% concordance with MYC amplification as detected by FISH. Immunohistochemistry for detection of vascular marker expression can facilitate characterization of poorly differentiated tumors with limited or absent vasoformative areas.	MYC amplification in >50% of postradiation angiosarcomas and a subset of nonradiation-associated angiosarcomas. Immunohistochemistry for c-myc shows nearly 100% concordance with MYC amplification as detected by FISH. Immunohistochemical detection of vascular markers can facilitate characterization of poorly differentiated tumors with limited or absent vasoformative areas.
Treatment	Total mastectomy; wide excision alone is associated with high recurrence rates. Radiotherapy and chemotherapy ineffective.	Total mastectomy; wide excision alone is associated with high recurrence rates. Radiotherapy and chemotherapy ineffective.
Clinical implication	Primary angiosarcoma, regardless of grade, has a poor prognosis with a mean survival of 1–2 y	Postradiation angiosarcoma, regardless of grade, has a poor prognosis with a mean survival of 1–2 y

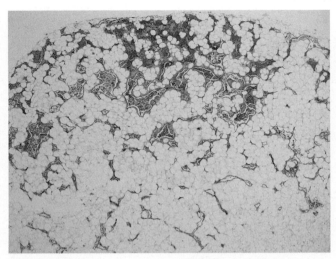

Figure 10.4.1   Postradiation angiosarcoma, showing diffuse infiltration of fat.

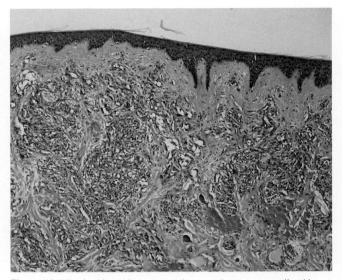

Figure 10.4.6   In this angiosarcoma, the vascular spaces are lined by multiple layers of enlarged, pleomorphic nuclei; note blood lakes.

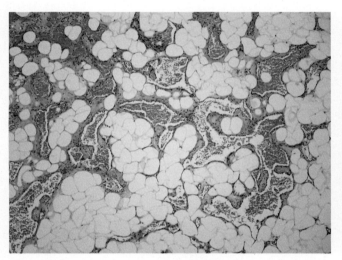

Figure 10.4.2   Complex, anastomosing, dilated vascular channels filled with erythrocytes are characteristic of postradiation angiosarcoma.

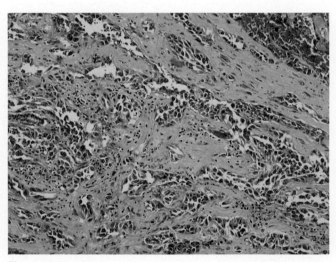

Figure 10.4.7   Extravasated erythrocytes are a common finding in high grade angiosarcoma.

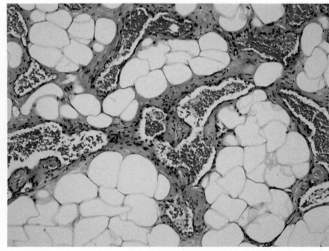

Figure 10.4.3   The vascular spaces are lined by a single layer of enlarged endothelial cells, without tufting.

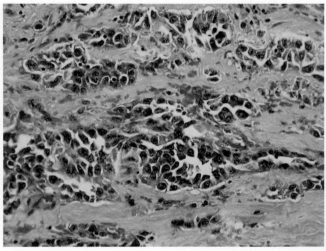

Figure 10.4.8   Multilayering of malignant endothelial cells may impart a solid growth pattern in some angiosarcomas.

10 Vascular Lesions

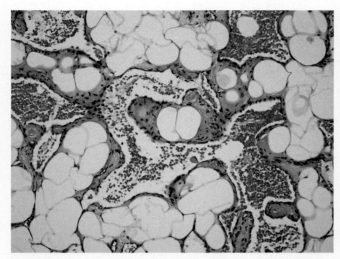

Figure 10.4.4   Anastomosing channels permeate fat in angiosarcoma.

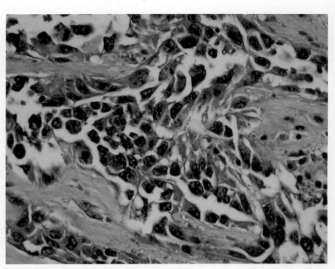

Figure 10.4.9   Primary angiosarcoma showing endothelial tufting and marked nuclear pleomorphism.

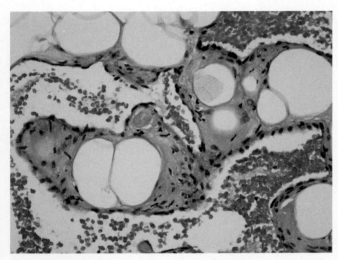

Figure 10.4.5   Plump nuclei bulge into the vascular lumens in postradiation angiosarcoma.

	Epithelioid Angiosarcoma	Poorly Differentiated Invasive Mammary Carcinoma
Age	Women over 50 y of age (approximately 20 y older than women with primary angiosarcoma). Most cases occur 2.5–11.5 y (median 4.5 y) after radiation therapy.	Adult women, often middle age or older
Location	Breast skin, frequently with extension into adjacent mammary parenchyma; may be extensive	Anywhere in the breast
Presentation	Multifocal, cutaneous, purple-blue and erythematous plaques, papules, or nodules within the field of radiation; frequently involves adjacent breast parenchyma; almost exclusively seen in patients with a history of radiation therapy	Mammographically detected mass, often interval cancers, or palpable mass
Imaging findings	None or skin thickening; associated ill-defined density with involvement of underlying breast parenchyma; MRI can be very useful in defining size.	Spiculated, solid mass on mammogram; taller than wide with irregular margins on ultrasound
Etiology	Radiation treatment for breast cancer	Unknown
Histology	1. Poorly-differentiated, infiltrative neoplasm with ill-defined cell borders, solid growth pattern, and epithelioid morphology resembling poorly differentiated carcinoma *(Figs. 10.5.1–10.5.4)* 2. Malignant cells have marked nuclear hyperchromasia and conspicuous mitotic activity, including atypical forms *(Fig. 10.5.4)* 3. "Epithelioid" endothelial cells have abundant amphophilic to eosinophilic cytoplasm and large vesicular nuclei *(Fig. 10.5.4)* 4. When the lesion involves the mammary parenchyma, solid islands of tumor infiltrate around or obliterate acinar structures *(Fig. 10.5.3)* 5. Vascular spaces, blood lakes, or slit-like spaces containing extravasated erythrocytes are often absent *(Figs. 10.5.3 and 10.5.4)* 6. Immunohistochemistry may be an important adjunct to demonstrate vascular differentiation *(Figs. 10.5.5–10.5.8)*	1. High combined histologic grade invasive mammary carcinoma of no special type *(Figs. 10.5.9–10.5.11)* 2. Solid growth pattern without gland formation *(Fig. 10.5.10)* 3. Large and pleomorphic nuclei *(Fig. 10.5.11)* 4. High mitotic rate *(Fig. 10.5.11)*
Special studies	MYC amplification in >50% of postradiation angiosarcomas; immunohistochemistry for c-myc shows nearly 100% concordance with MYC amplification as detected by FISH. Since poorly differentiated angiosarcomas may demonstrate limited expression of endothelial cell markers, use of a battery of markers (Factor VIII, CD31, CD34, D2-40, and FLI-1) is often necessary.	Strong and diffuse cytokeratin expression distinguishes from angiosarcoma; subset may be CK7 and/or GATA3 negative; often triple negative (ER–, PR–, HER2–); negative for endothelial markers

	Epithelioid Angiosarcoma	Poorly Differentiated Invasive Mammary Carcinoma
	Expression of cytokeratin (CAM5.2 and AE1/AE3) and EMA have been reported in up to 50% of epithelioid angiosarcomas, leading to a misdiagnosis of carcinoma.	
Treatment	Total mastectomy; wide excision alone is associated with high recurrence rates. Radiotherapy and chemotherapy ineffective.	Neoadjuvant chemotherapy followed by lumpectomy or mastectomy and axillary lymph node evaluation; ± radiation therapy
Clinical implication	Postradiation epithelioid angiosarcoma, regardless of grade, has a poor prognosis with a mean survival of 1–2 y	Approximately 35% recurrence rate, most occurring the first 5 y following diagnosis

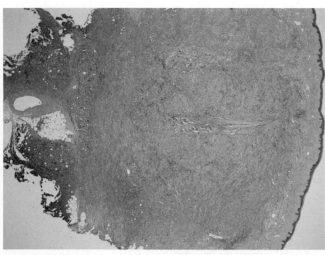

Figure 10.5.1 In this postradiation epithelioid angiosarcoma, the skin and adjacent breast parenchyma are infiltrated by a solid neoplastic proliferation.

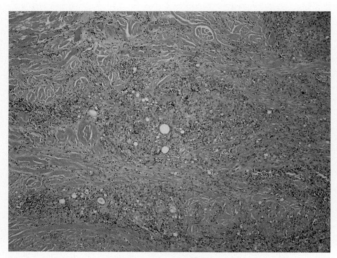

Figure 10.5.2 Epithelioid angiosaroma infiltrates dermal collagen. Obvious vasoformative areas are lacking.

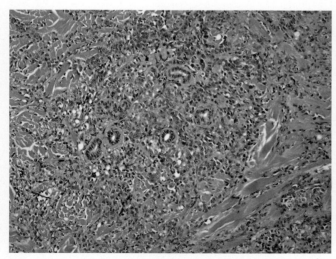

Figure 10.5.3 Lobular units and adjacent nonspecialized connective tissue are infiltrated by epithelioid angiosarcoma.

Figure 10.5.9 Invasive mammary carcinoma, of no special type, showing solid nests of malignant epithelial cells.

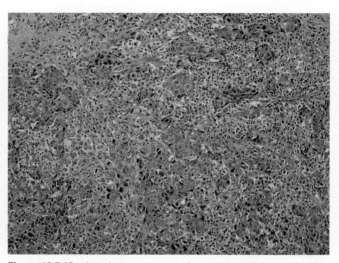

Figure 10.5.10 Invasive mammary carcinoma, no special type, showing a high combined histologic grade.

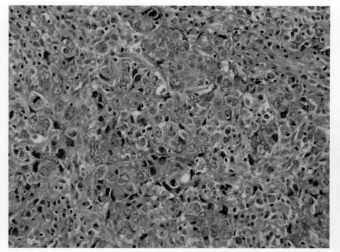

Figure 10.5.11 Nest of malignant epithelial cells and frequent mitotic figures are characteristic of invasive mammary carcinoma of no special type, having a high combined histologic grade.

10 Vascular Lesions

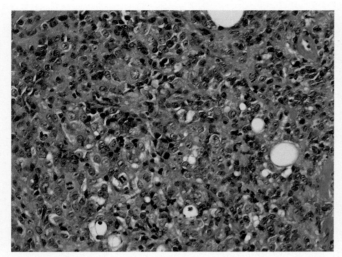

Figure 10.5.4   In epithelioid angiosarcoma, the malignant cells have a solid growth pattern, cytologic features of malignant epithelium, and frequent mitoses.

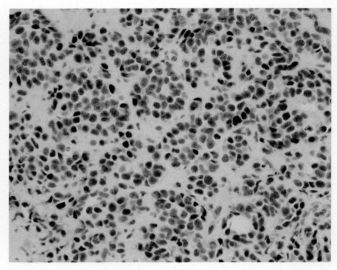

Figure 10.5.7   Nuclear expression of FLI-1 is a sensitive marker for angiosarcoma.

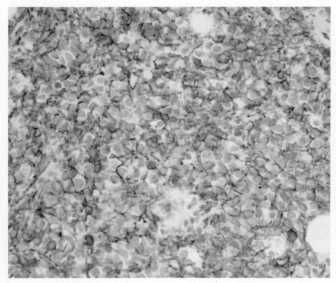

Figure 10.5.5   An immunohistochemical study using antibodies to CD31 shows strong membranous expression in epithelioid angiosarcoma.

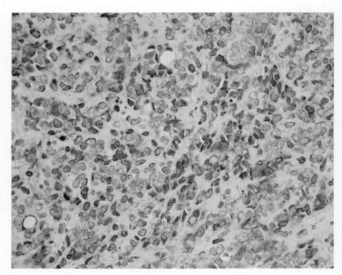

Figure 10.5.8   Cytoplasmic expression of D2-40 by epithelioid angiosarcoma.

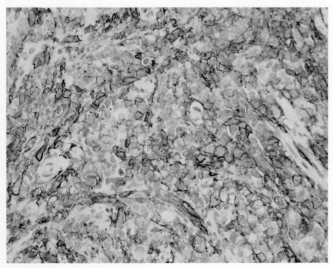

Figure 10.5.6   Epithelioid angiosarcoma shows strong, membranous expression of CD34.

SUGGESTED READINGS

Billings SD, McKenney JK, Folpe AL, et al. Cutaneous angiosarcoma following breast-conserving surgery and radiation: an analysis of 27 cases. *Am J Surg Pathol.* 2004;28:781–788.

Brenn T, Fletcher CD. Postradiation vascular proliferations: an increasing problem. *Histopathology.* 2006;48:106–114.

Brenn T, Fletcher CD. Radiation-associated cutaneous atypical vascular lesions and angiosarcoma: clinicopathologic analysis of 42 cases. *Am J Surg Pathol.* 2005;29:983–996.

Fineberg S, Rosen PP. Cutaneous angiosarcoma and atypical vascular lesions of the skin and breast after radiation therapy for breast carcinoma. *Am J Clin Pathol.* 1994;102:757–763.

Folpe AL, Chand EM, Goldblum JR, et al. Expression of Fli-1, a nuclear transcription factor, distinguishes vascular neoplasms from potential mimics. *Am J Surg Pathol.* 2001;25:1061–1066.

Kryvenko ON, Chitale DA, VanEgmond EM, et al. Angiolipoma of the female breast: clinicomorphological correlation of 52 cases. *Int J Surg Pathol.* 2011;19:35–43.

Lakhani SR, Ellis IO, Schnitt SJ, et al., ed. *WHO Classification of Tumors of the Breast.* 4 ed. Lyon: IARC; 2012.

Lucas DR. Angiosarcoma, radiation-associated angiosarcoma, and atypical vascular lesion. *Archiv Pathol Lab Med.* 2009;133:1804–1809.

Monroe AT, Feigenberg SJ, Mendenhall NP. Angiosarcoma after breast-conserving therapy. *Cancer.* 2003;97:1832–1840.

Nascimento AF, Raut CP, Fletcher CD. Primary angiosarcoma of the breast: clinicopathologic analysis of 49 cases, suggesting that grade is not prognostic. *Am J Surg Pathol.* 2008;32:1896–1904.

Patton KT, Deyrup AT, Weiss SW. Atypical vascular lesions after surgery and radiation of the breast: a clinicopathologic study of 32 cases analyzing histologic heterogeneity and association with angiosarcoma. *Am J Surg Pathol.* 2008;32:943–950.

Requena L, Kutzner H, Mentzel T, et al. Benign vascular proliferations in irradiated skin. *Am J Surg Pathol.* 2002;26:328–37.

Rosen PP, Kimmel M, Ernsberger D. Mammary angiosarcoma. The prognostic significance of tumor differentiation. *Cancer.* 1988;62:2145–2151.

Rosen PP, Ridolfi RL. The perilobular hemangioma. A benign microscopic vascular lesion of the breast. *Am J Clin Pathol.* 1977;68:21–23.

Schnitt SJ. Angiosarcoma of the mammary skin following conservative surgery and radiation therapy for breast cancer. *Pathol Case Rev.* 1999;4:194–198.

Vorburger SA, Xing Y, Hunt KK, et al. Angiosarcoma of the breast. *Cancer.* 2005;104:2682–2688.

Yap J, Chuba PJ, Thomas R, et al. Sarcoma as a second malignancy after treatment for breast cancer. *Int J Radiat Oncol Biol Phys.* 2002;52:1231–1237.

10 Vascular Lesions

11

Male Breast

	Florid-Phase Gynecomastia	Atypical Ductal Hyperplasia (ADH) in Gynecomastia
Age	Adolescent boys and men in sixth and seventh decade, newborns (rare)	Late teens and adults
Location	Unilateral or bilateral, central and retroareolar	Central, retroareolar
Presentation	Unilateral or bilateral breast mass(es)	Rarely encountered in breast specimens from males with long-standing gynecomastia
Imaging Findings	Nodular density by mammography; ultrasound shows avascular, hypoechoic, nodular or poorly defined density parallel to the chest wall, without posterior enhancement or shadowing	Nodular density by mammography; on ultrasound, avascular, hypoechoic, nodular or poorly defined density parallel to the chest wall, without posterior enhancement or shadowing
Etiology	Relative or absolute estrogen excess: (1) therapeutic estrogen administration for treatment of prostate cancer; (2) increased endogenous production by tumors (e.g., Leydig cell tumor); (3) increased aromatization of androgens to estrogens (e.g., alcoholic cirrhosis, obesity and aging); (4) altered androgen to estrogen ratio (cirrhosis, renal failure, puberty, aging, anabolic steroids); (5) drugs decreasing androgen action, including illicit drugs; (6) transient exposure of male infants to maternal hormones	Unknown; often associated with gynecomastia, but etiologic factors leading to the specific development of ADH within gynecomastia are not known
Histology	1. Increased number of ducts within fibrous stroma with periductal edema and myxoid stroma *(Fig. 11.1.1)* 2. Hyperplasia in ducts with thin, tapering micropapillae composed of cells with scant cytoplasm and pyknotic nuclei *(Figs. 11.1.1–11.1.3)* 3. Epithelial micropapillae composed of cells that appear "stuck" to underlying luminal epithelium, rather than emanating from basement membrane *(Figs. 11.1.3 and 11.1.4)* 4. Individual cell placement irregular and cell borders indistinct *(Fig. 11.1.4)* 5. Stroma frequently resembles pseudoangiomatous stromal hyperplasia	1. Ducts are partially involved by a uniform population of bland cells; partial involvement is essential for diagnosis because lobular units are (usually) not present in male breast tissue *(Figs. 11.1.5 and 11.1.6)* 2. Cells are evenly placed and secondary spaces are rigid with formation of microrosettes *(Figs. 11.1.7 and 11.1.8)* 3. Residual, normally polarized epithelium is present at the periphery of a portion of the duct *(Fig. 11.1.8)*
Special Studies	None	None

	Florid-Phase Gynecomastia	**Atypical Ductal Hyperplasia (ADH) in Gynecomastia**
Treatment	None, usually resolves; excision if cosmetically disfiguring	Total mastectomy
Clinical implication	None, no association with subsequent cancer risk	Due to rarity, clinical implications are not known; however, mastectomy is curative and the usual approach

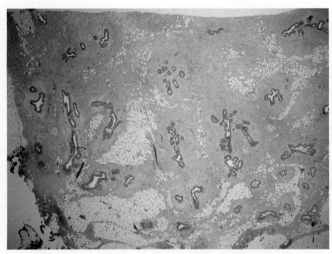

Figure 11.1.1   Gynectomastia: Many ducts are expanded by an epithelial proliferation, and are encircled by dense stroma.

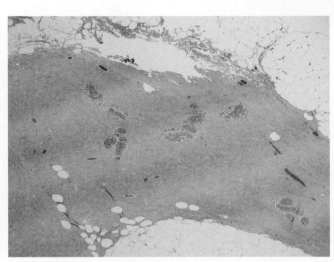

Figure 11.1.5   Several ducts are expanded by an epithelial proliferation in ADH.

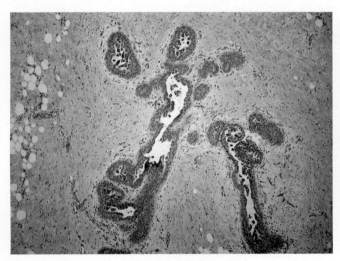

Figure 11.1.2   Florid hyperplasia of gynecomastia, showing numerous micropapillae.

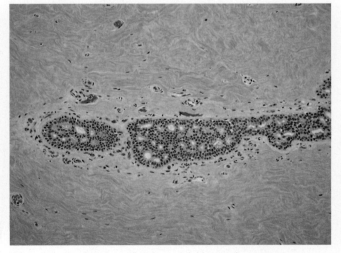

Figure 11.1.6   Cellular uniformity and rigid secondary spaces are present. Some secondary spaces are slit-like, and a normal cell population is present peripherally in this example of ADH.

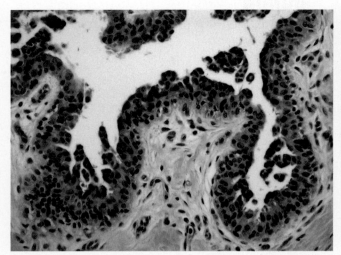

Figure 11.1.3 The micropapillae of gynecomastia are thin and tapering, and are composed of cells with pyknotic nuclei.

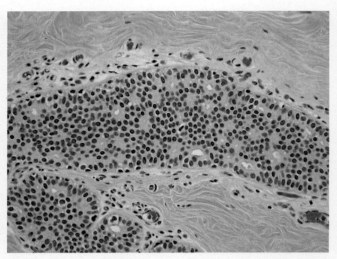

Figure 11.1.7 ADH showing some irregular secondary spaces and residual normal epithelium.

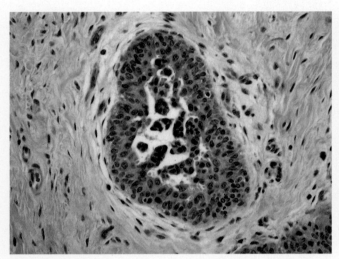

Figure 11.1.4 The micropapillae of gynectomastia appear "stuck" on the luminal epithelium, rather than extending from the basement membrane.

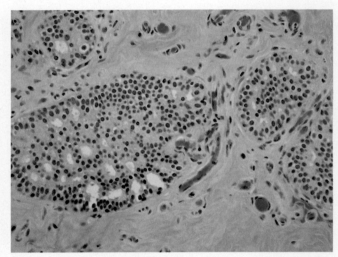

Figure 11.1.8 While some microrosettes are present, other secondary spaces are irregular in ADH.

	ADH	Low-Grade Ductal Carcinoma In Situ (DCIS)
Age	Late teens and adults	Adult males
Location	Central, retroareolar	Central, retroareolar
Presentation	Rarely encountered in breast specimens from males with long-standing gynecomastia	Rare finding in breast specimens in men with long-standing gynecomastia; less commonly palpable mass or bloody nipple discharge
Imaging findings	Same as in gynecomastia. Nodular density by mammography; on ultrasound, avascular, hypoechoic, nodular or poorly defined density parallel to the chest wall without posterior enhancement or shadowing.	None specific enough to distinguish from gynecomastia; nodular density by mammography; ultrasound shows avascular, hypoechoic, nodular or poorly defined density parallel to the chest wall, without posterior enhancement or shadowing; rarely associated with calcification
Etiology	Unknown; often associated with gynecomastia, but etiologic factors leading to the specific development of ADH within gynecomastia are not known	Unknown
Histology	1. Ducts are partially involved by a uniform population of bland cells; partial involvement is essential for diagnosis because lobular units are (usually) not present in male breast tissue *(Figs. 11.2.1–11.2.4)* 2. Cells are evenly placed and secondary spaces are rigid, with formation of microrosettes, although irregular secondary spaces remain *(Fig. 11.2.3)* 3. Residual, normally polarized epithelium is present at the periphery of a portion of the duct *(Fig. 11.2.4)*	1. Extensive process; multiple ducts show distention and distortion by a uniform epithelial proliferation *(Fig. 11.2.5)* 2. Usually low or intermediate grade, and often solid growth pattern with microrosette formation *(Figs. 11.2.6–11.2.8)*
Special studies	None	Immunohistochemical evaluation of hormone receptor status, as performed for female ductal carcinoma is appropriate
Treatment	Total mastectomy	Total mastectomy
Clinical implication	Due to rarity, clinical implications are not known; however, mastectomy is curative and the usual approach	Total mastectomy is curative

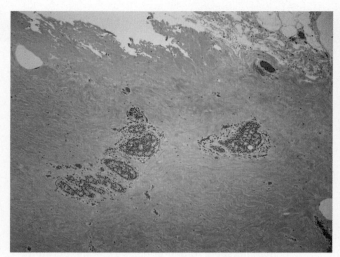

Figure 11.2.1   Several ducts are partially expanded by a cellular proliferation with cribriform architecture in ADH.

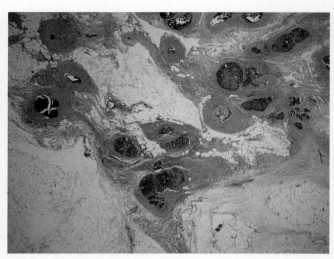

Figure 11.2.5   Ducts are greatly distorted by an epithelial proliferation
in this example of DCIS.

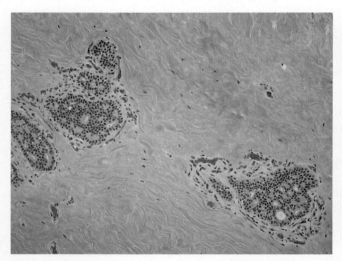

Figure 11.2.2   There is a normal population of cells present peripherally
in these ducts with ADH.

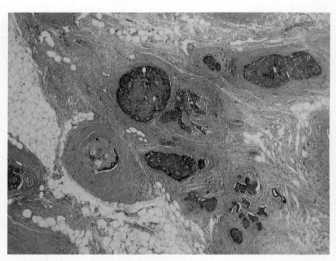

Figure 11.2.6   Characteristic of DCIS, these ducts are distended by an
epithelial proliferation having a solid growth pattern.

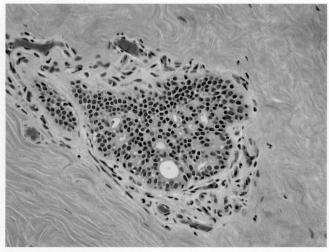

Figure 11.2.3   Some of the secondary spaces are crisp, but others are
irregular, supporting the diagnosis of ADH.

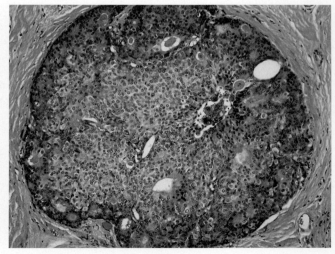

Figure 11.2.7   Although there is a suggestion of irregular secondary
spaces, the degree of cellular proliferation and cellular uniformity requires a diagnosis of DCIS.

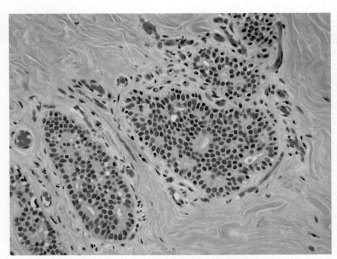

Figure 11.2.4   Centrally, there is a uniform population of bland cells in this example of ADH. Note normal polarity at periphery and some irregular secondary spaces.

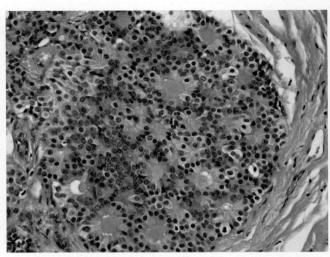

Figure 11.2.8   Well-formed microrosettes are present in this example of DCIS.

11.3

SOLID-PATTERN DUCTAL CARCINOMA IN SITU IN A PAPILLOMA VS. INVASIVE MAMMARY CARCINOMA WITH NODULAR PATTERN (SUGGESTING ORIGIN FROM PAPILLOMAS)

	Solid-Pattern DCIS in a Papilloma	Invasive Mammary Carcinoma with Nodular Pattern (Suggesting Origin from Papillomas)
Age	Adult males	Adult males
Location	Central, retroareolar	Central, retroareolar
Presentation	Most commonly a subareolar palpable nodule	Most commonly a palpable, firm, irregular subareolar nodule
Imaging findings	Nodular density; irregular mass with microlobulated margins on ultrasound	Irregular subareolar mass with spiculations or indistinct margins by mammography; ultrasound shows irregular mass with microlobulated margins
Etiology	Unknown	Unknown
Histology	1. Circumscribed, encysted nodule consisting of a solid, uniform epithelial proliferation *(Fig. 11.3.1)* 2. Fibrovascular cores may be subtle *(Fig. 11.3.2)* 3. Residual duct wall lining may not be obvious *(Fig. 11.3.3)* 4. Neoplastic proliferation usually has low- or intermediate-grade nuclei *(Fig. 11.3.4)* 5. Linearly arranged neoplastic epithelium associated with hemosiderin may mimic invasion *(Fig. 11.3.4)*	1. Expansile mass with nodules extending into fat *(Figs. 11.3.5–11.3.7)* 2. Absence of delimiting fibrous duct wall *(Fig. 11.3.6)* 3. Solid growth pattern composed of cells with intermediate- or high-grade nuclei *(Fig. 11.3.7)*
Special studies	None; myoepithelial cells when present may be useful in delineating fibrovascular cores or residual duct lining; their absence does not equate to invasive carcinoma	Assessment of hormone receptors *(Fig. 11.3.8)* and HER2 status, as performed for female breast cancer, is appropriate
Treatment	Total mastectomy	Total mastectomy, sentinel lymph node mapping, and chemotherapy (depending on stage and ancillary test results)
Clinical implication	Mastectomy is curative	Survival based on stage, similar to that of stage-matched women with invasive breast carcinoma

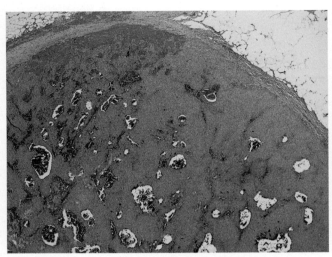

Figure 11.3.1   Solid pattern DCIS involving an intraductal papilloma. Note sharply circumscribed growth pattern and presence of fibrovascular cores.

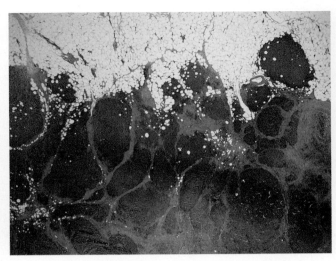

Figure 11.3.5   Expansile nodules of invasive carcinoma show an irregular interface with adjacent fat in this example of invasive mammary carcinoma of no special type.

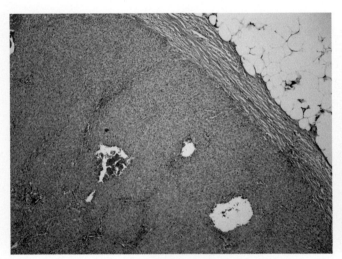

Figure 11.3.2   Encysting fibrous duct wall sharply delimits the neoplastic proliferation of DCIS cells within an intraductal papilloma.

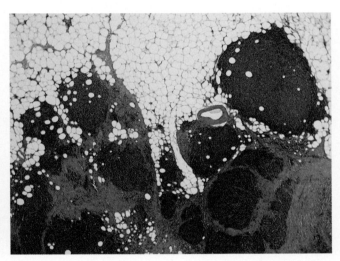

Figure 11.3.6   Invasive mammary carcinoma (no special type): Multiple infiltrative nests extend into the fat.

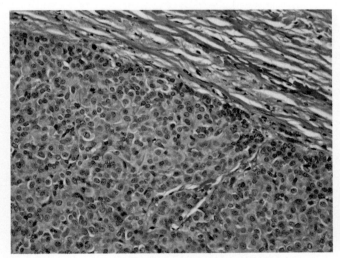

Figure 11.3.3   Low-grade nuclei are characteristic of DCIS involving an intraductal papilloma in men.

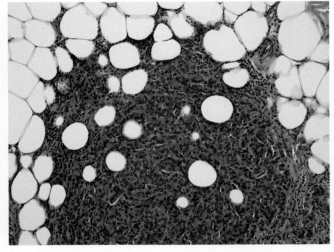

Figure 11.3.7   Invasive mammary carcinomas in men are graded using the modified Nottingham grading system; this example has an intermediate (Grade 2) combined histologic grade.

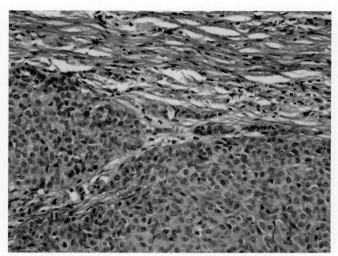

Figure 11.3.4   A few tumor cell nests are present in the encysting fibrous tissue, but these are associated with hemosiderin, and have a linear arrangement, indicative of entrapment and not invasion.

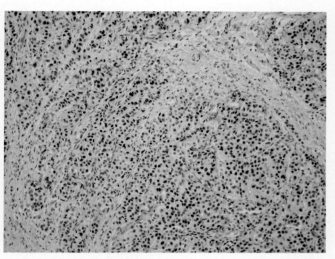

Figure 11.3.8   Strong expression of estrogen receptor by this invasive carcinoma of no special type is characteristic of more than 90% of male breast cancers. Hormone receptor analysis and HER2 assessment should be performed on all invasive carcinomas in males.

SUGGESTED READINGS

Anderson WF, Devesa SS. In situ male breast carcinoma in the surveillance, epidemiology, and end results database of the National Cancer Institute. *Cancer.* 2005;104:1733–1741.

Bannayan GA, Hajdu SI. Gynecomastia: clinicopathologic study of 351 cases. *Am J Clin Pathol.* 1972;57:431–437.

Camus MG, Joshi MG, Mackarem G, et al. Ductal carcinoma in situ of the male breast. *Cancer.* 1994;74:1289–1293.

Hittmair AP, Lininger RA, Tavassoli FA. Ductal carcinoma in situ (DCIS) in the male breast: a morphologic study of 84 cases of pure DCIS and 30 cases of DCIS associated with invasive carcinoma--a preliminary report. *Cancer.* 1998;83:2139–2149.

Joshi MG, Lee AK, Loda M, et al. Male breast carcinoma: an evaluation of prognostic factors contributing to a poorer outcome. *Cancer.* 1996;77:490–498.

Lapid O, Jolink F, Meijer SL. Pathological findings in gynecomastia: analysis of 5113 breasts. *Ann Plast Surg.* 2013;74(2):163–166.

Pant K, Dutta U. Understanding and management of male breast cancer: a critical review. *Med Oncol.* 2008;25:294–298.

11 Male Breast

Index